MW00977618

LifeMaps for Midlife Women

How Do You Say No to Depression, No to Ailments, and Yes to Sex?

By

Linda Hughes, Ed.D.

This book is a work of non-fiction. Names and places have been changed to protect the privacy of all individuals. The events and situations are true.

ISBN: 1-4107-9604-3 (e-book)
ISBN: 1-4107-9603-5 (Paperback)

This book is printed on acid free paper.

1stBooks - rev. 12/08/03

Acknowledgements

My heartfelt appreciation goes out to the hundreds of thousands of women in North America and thirteen other countries who have attended my seminars and speeches, and all of those I've met during my personal travels around the world. These are your stories, your insights, and your inspirations. Thank you all.

The women who volunteered to participate in my research study on midlife women deserve kudos for their willingness to candidly share their stories about the good and bad aspects of being middle aged. Their names have been changed in order to protect their privacy, but their agreement to let their stories be told allows us to learn from their experiences.

I am also grateful to my instructors and fellow classmates at the University of Georgia who were so generous in contributing suggestions, critiques, and support for this work. I always felt privileged to be in the midst of so many brilliant and caring people.

Finally, I am deeply indebted to Dr. Sharan Merriam, my advisor at UGA. Without fail, every time I'd write up a piece of research about midlife women, she'd give it back, telling me to do more and do it better. In the end, no stone was left unturned. Thank you, Dr. Merriam, for making me give my best. Although my original intent had been to study other women, you made it a journey of self-discovery as well.

Dedication

LifeMaps for Midlife Women is dedicated to all of you women out there who are seeking answers to questions about this time of life called midlife. May this book be just the beginning of your exciting journey of self-discovery, exploration, and celebration of this, the best time of life.

Table of Contents

Introduction

"One is not born, but rather becomes, a woman."
Simone de Beauvoir (1949)

The fact that you're reading this means there's a good chance you're one of the 37 million Baby Boomer women between the ages of 40 - 60 who wants to know what on earth to do with this new phase of life, this midlife thing. You've undoubtedly heard countless stories about what it's like to make the shocking discovery that you're no longer young, stories about reaching back to swipe off something stuck to your butt and then realizing that it *is* your butt, about being called the dreaded "ma'am" for the first time, and about unexpectedly passing a mirror and seeing your mother. In my case, it was looking at an old photo of my *grandmother* and being dumbstruck upon realizing that, if I had my hair in a bun, that's *me*!

In our misguidedly youth-oriented culture, aging can be scary. On the other hand, when we use our years of experience and acquired wisdom to create our own life journeys, our own LifeMaps, midlife can be the most *exquisite* time of life.

You might be saying, "That's not what I've heard!" Well, a lot of what you've heard is just plumb wrong.

1

Linda Hughes, Ed.D.

Midlife Myths and Realities

The first thing this book does is dispel popular myths about midlife. For instance, the media too often makes it seem as if all midlife women are alike, with the same family experiences, aging concerns, and blasé interests. Not true. We've been unique individuals all of our lives and will be until we push up daisies. Another myth, if you believe advertisements, is that hot flashes attack most menopausal women. No. Medical research reveals that the majority of menopausal women are as cool as a cucumber. Likewise, you might think that sexual desire goes caput as we age. Ha! Wait until you read the stories about women who are hot all right, but for sex! You might even have fallen for the notion that all older women are supposed to be domestic, cooking up Martha-Stewart-style meals. Not so. I know a fifty-five-year-old who got rid of her stove so that everyone would stop expecting her to feed them. And, you might believe the jokes about mental ability taking a dive in middle age with "old timers' disease." Nope. Research proves that's not true, either.

Of course, there are some disturbing truths that midlife women must face, like negative media images, unflattering stereotypes, ageism, sexism, and work and wage inequities. This book helps you face those real issues head-on, as well as dealing with the plethora of myths. To help you deal with the myths, you'll work with a list of things that we need to let go of in midlife versus things that we can embrace, like fantasy vs. reality, blind faith vs. enlightened faith, and wishful thinking vs. actionable planning.

There are many expectations and fantasies that we grew up with that never have done us any good. (Have *you* seen the prince lately? Would you want him if you did?) When we're first whacked with the startling fact that our lives are at least half over, most of us panic. But once we catch our breaths, we settle down and resolve not to waste one more minute on unrealistic expectations and stupid fantasies. It's time to get real and enjoy real life.

What's a LifeMap?

In order to get real, you can use this book to create your own LifeMap, a soul system, something like a solar system, which puts the many aspects of your life into focus and balance. It's common in our culture for us to think in terms of following a flat, linear path: set a goal and then take the necessary steps to get to it. But our lives aren't neat flat paths any more than the earth is flat. We don't just have goals; we have needs and desires, talents and abilities, and wisdom and experience. Our lives are complex, twirling systems with our souls in the center, lots of planets on different orbital paths, an occasional meteor crashing into everything, a sky awash in scintillating stars, and, of course, the inevitable alien (usually a relative or co-worker) popping in to keep things a little wacko.

There are seven areas, planets if you will, of our lives that we need to attend to in order to keep our lives in balance. That balance allows us to be whole and enjoy ourselves to the fullest. We've always needed to attend to these seven areas, but most of us didn't because we were busy trying to be Barbie dolls, pleasing others (some who didn't deserve to be pleased), and searching for meaning in the world while missing the meaning that already dwelt within us. So, here we are at midlife, finally ready to attend to those things that we've been ignoring, the areas of life that are at this very moment, as it turns out, screaming for our attention. Just listen to yourself and you'll hear what they are.

The seven areas included in LifeMaps are: body, mind, relationships, work, money, space, and spirituality. In my twenty years of conducting workshops for hundreds of thousands of women around the world, these are the areas of life that I've learned are most important to women. Because I am a midlife woman and because of my research about midlife women for my doctorate degree, the LifeMaps concept has evolved over the years to specifically address the needs of midlife women. But, as you'll see, LifeMaps can be used to address the needs of anyone at any age.

Are you ready to move beyond the craziness of youth? Ready to focus on those areas that need attention so that you can allow your soul system to float in balance? Are you ready to embrace your whole being so that you can enjoy midlife and beyond? If so, you're ready to create your own midlife LifeMap. There are activities in each chapter so that you can chart out a map for an unparalleled life adventure that is yours and yours alone.

While creating your LifeMap, it's possible you'll rediscover parts of yourself that were long ago banished into outer space. For example, you'll have a chance to bring back that wild child that you once were, the girl that felt no fear and no limitations. Most women find this to be exhilarating! It's also likely that you'll experience new insights. Participating in discussion groups with other women having similar experiences can be very helpful in deciding what to do with this new knowledge. I encourage you to share your LifeMap experience with others, if you choose to do so.

After creating your LifeMap, you'll be able to see what parts of your life are doing well and what parts need work or play. You'll have a vision for what you want to do differently and will be inspired to do it.

In the future you'll be able to recreate your map from time-to-time to meet your changing needs. Your soul system is gliding through space and expanding as surely as is our solar system. It makes sense to readjust your course every now and then.

Let me suggest that you do what I do when I work with my own LifeMap: Skip the parts that don't grab your attention, concentrate on what speaks to you most right now, and later fit in the rest. Use the references cited throughout the book and listed in the back to help you learn more about whatever peaks your interest. It's your universe and you can create it to be any way that you want it to be.

So, soar on in and enjoy your LifeMap. It'll help you enjoy your life!

Linda Hughes, Ed.D.

Chapter 1 ~ Create Your LifeMap, Create Your Life

"Anyone can fly.
All you need is somewhere to go that you can't get to any other way.
The next thing you know, you're flying among the stars."
Faith Ringgold (1996)

There were about two hundred women in the audience on the day that the concept of LifeMaps was born. I was in the middle of my most popular seminar at that time, *TrailBlazers,* a program I'd worked long and hard to develop, one that I'd presented a hundred times. The idea was that we follow a path in life and always come to a fork in the road, forcing a decision as to which way to go. Our choice is never a mistake because, even if we take a wrong turn, we eventually figure out it was a poor choice, which motivates us to find a way to a smoother path. My audiences, who consistently rated my programs and me amongst the top in my field, had always received this concept very well. I had audiotapes to go with the program, the workbook was attractive, and the Power Point illustrations were dazzling. I even used the old Roy Rogers tune, *Happy Trails*, to open and close the soiree. The program was honed to perfection.

Linda Hughes, Ed.D.

On that day, however, I looked out at the sea of shining faces and suddenly knew that using an example of a flat trail was too limiting for these women. Their lives, and mine, are much more complicated than that. Right then and there, I stopped what I was saying and looked at the charming picture of a trail on the screen. Silence hung in the air for a few measured moments, and then I said, "This is a nice idea, but do any of you have lives that are this simple and neat?" At first I heard a few no answers but after considering the question many more said, "No!"

"What about a solar system?" I asked, struck with a memory of a seminar I'd attended many years earlier by Dr. Milt Cudney of Western Michigan University. He'd said that each of our lives is a unique universe. As that concept evolved through the discussion at my seminar, I knew that this is much more representative of women's lives than a flat trail. (Although one woman insisted that her life is a cosmic wormhole.)

Others throughout history have envisioned life in ways different from a linear progression. Many have seen it as a circle, a belief that is illustrated in the ancient Sanskrit Mandala circles [1], Celtic circles of stones [2], and the Native American perception of the sacred circle of life [3]. Yet others think of life as a web. William Shakespeare said, "The web of our life is of a mingled yarn" [4]; Frances Hesselbein, former director of the International Girl Scouts, writes about managing in a round world [5]; and many researchers report that their subjects describe life as a circle, web, or cyclical

8

pattern [6-11]. So, the notion that our lives aren't well represented by a flat line isn't new. If we take these concepts and add movement, space, and color, we have a solar system. All of these thoughts jousted in my head on that day when I spontaneously decided to change my whole seminar while I was right in the middle of a seminar.

The Soul System

Each of our lives consists of a center, a soul, and many facets of life that are like planets, moons, meteors, asteroids, satellites, and UFOs circling around and in and out of our soul area. We reach out to grasp what we need, sometimes missing as it eludes us, only to try again the next time it orbits close-by.

Like any solar system, this one hangs in precarious balance, needing all of its elements in order to stay afloat and not explode into shards that career off into outer space or implode into a black hole. All of the pieces are necessary in order for the system to stay whole. Thus, we're constantly doing a balancing act, keeping all of the facets of our lives in motion. We don't follow a road, arrive somewhere, and then we're done. Instead, our lives are always moving through space and expanding, like quantum physics suppositions that the universe moves and expands, giving us endless opportunities for new experiences, any of which can bring us sorrow or joy. Our aim is to keep the sorrow from dominating our systems so that we can expand our lives enough to move into new space where we're more likely to run into and clasp onto new options for reveling in life's moments of sheer joy.

Now, by midlife, we're aware of this need for balance because we've been so busy and out of balance for so long. We each have our own way of thinking about it - you might think of it as multi-tasking, getting involved, or going crazy – but, however you label it, I'm asking that you suspend your present beliefs, at least for a little while, and envision a glittering, twirling, 3-dimensional, soul system in which balance represents wholeness. That's what happens when you get clear about what matters in your life and clear out the rest. It's like cleaning out the space junk so that you have room to view the glory of your existence.

Join Your Soul System and Your LifeMap

This book will help you see what it is that you need to do in order to bring balance, wholeness, and joy into your life. You'll map out your life journey by adding to your LifeMap after reading each chapter and writing down your thoughts regarding each of the seven areas of life – body, mind, relationships, work, money, space, and spirituality. Although there's no way here to represent your LifeMap's soul system except on flat paper, you can imagine it with depth, color, and movement. It isn't possible for all of these areas of life to be in perfect balance at all times, but it is possible to keep them in sight and attend to them as soon as possible.

Although LifeMapping is an important task, it isn't tattooed onto your forehead. You can easily change it as you change your life. Begin the process by answering the questions and doing the activities on the next couple of pages. Although you'll work on your map while you read this book, you can continue to write your thoughts for months and years to come. It's a life-long learning process that can change your life for the rest of your life.

Begin LifeMapping

1. Look at page 15. This is a basic version of a LifeMap.

2. On the LifeMap, draw a line from your inner soul circle to each circle that you genuinely feel is connected to you. The following questions will help. If you answer "yes" to a question, draw a line between your soul circle and the outer circle for that question. If you answer "no," there's no connection, so don't draw a line. If you're not sure, a dotted or squiggly line might be appropriate.

   a. Body: *Do I take care of my body so that it can be healthy? Do I eat pretty well and exercise at least moderately?*

   b. Mind: *Do I "feed my mind," allowing myself to learn and consider new options? Am I relatively mentally healthy?*

   c. Relationships: *Are my primary relationships satisfying? Do they contribute to my well-being and the well-being of others?*

   d. Work: *Is my work satisfying, even if only for the reason that it gives me other things in life that I want, like an income and stability? Do I go to work on most days without feeling dread?*

   e. Money: *Do I know how much money I'll need for retirement? Am I prepared for my financial future?*

    f. Space: *Do I have a place in my home or spot outdoors where I can meditate, pray, read, do anything I choose, or do nothing at all?*

    g. Spirituality: *Am I clear with myself about what spirituality means to me? Do I feel spiritually fulfilled?*

3. How many lines did you draw? _____

   Are you happy with that number? _____

4. Write down each life area (outer circle) where there was no line or a line that isn't straight.

   _____

   _____

   _____

   _____

5. These are the areas of your life that need the most work. Begin with and concentrate on these areas as you read this book. (There's a chapter for each area.) If you connected to every area with a solid, straight line that means your life might be wonderfully balanced. But read on anyway just in case you're living in la-la land and need to come down to earth. Are there no lines on your map? That means every area needs work, so you can begin anywhere you choose!

6. You now have the beginnings of your own personal LifeMap, which already illustrates which areas of your life are okay and which aren't so great. Don't worry if you can't decide what to

do with your L*ife*M*ap* at this point. The following chapters will help you fill it in as you go.

Your LifeMap

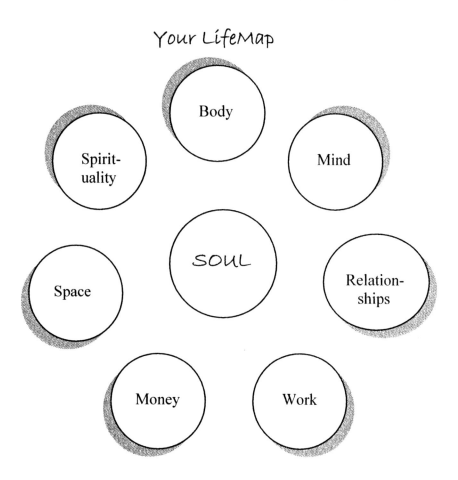

Draw a line from your Soul Center to each area of your
life that you feel connected to.
If you're not sure, a dotted or squiggly line might
represent how you feel.
If there is no line, no connection, that's an area you need
to begin to work on.

Chapter 2 ~ The Truth About Those Nasty Midlife Myths

"It's hard to feel middle-aged,
because how can you tell how long you are going to live?"
Mignon McLaughlin (1963)

Aging is a natural part of life. If you're not doing it, you're dead. We age throughout our entire lives, so to think of aging as something that only happens to a person after forty or fifty years is ridiculous. The changes in our bodies and minds between the ages of 11 and 14 when we were going through puberty are no more or less profound than those between the ages of 51 and 54. Yet, in North American youth-oriented culture (this doesn't happen in all cultures), aging is treated like a failure on the part of the woman who deigns to do it.

Of course, that attitude is lame-brained. But with that kind of mind-set hanging around, it's no wonder that some women balk at the thought of aging. When we look at all of the popular myths about midlife, it's easy to see how intentional and unintentional misinformation is publicly circulated and comes to be believed as the truth.

Sometimes the inaccurate information is conjured up in order to nurture and prey upon the fears of midlife women, impelling us to buy consumer goods. No one has a greater investment in our insecurities than advertisers and the companies they represent. If we didn't fear aging, we wouldn't buy so many anti-aging products. We can handle that by facing our fears, so that no matter what advertisers try to make us believe, we'll know better than to fall for their hype.

Sometimes the intention is to keep us from realizing the social, professional, and political power that we could wield as a group, seeing that we're nearly 14% of the population and it's estimated that we'll be the largest demographic group in the nation by 2008 [12]. We're told to vote this way or that and believe this or that with the assumption that we don't know enough to make our own decisions. We can handle that by making clear, informed, socially responsible decisions on our own, regardless of what anyone else tells us we should be doing.

And, sometimes we ourselves unintentionally propagate midlife myths simply by believing them and passing them along as the gospel truth. A woman recently told me that women in middle age grow cellulite cells on their shoulders. Once I managed to close my dropped jaw, I asked where she'd heard that. She said, "Everyone knows that." When I asked, "Who is 'everyone'?" she muttered and scurried away. Check your shoulders. Got saddlebags up there? No. This is just another midlife myth, one probably initiated by someone trying to scare women into buying a product. No more!

The following discussion about three major midlife myths allows us to deal with facts rather than fiction. Of course, hard, cold facts aren't always comforting, so there are also some touching and humorous real life stories that I've heard from women in my seminars and research study. And, there are LifeMap activities that will help you clarify your thinking regarding your aging process so that you'll be better able to accept aging as the natural part of life that it is.

You're probably familiar with these urban myths of midlife because, if you're like most of us, you've believed some of them. As you read, note which ones you thought were true.

Midlife Myth #1:

Midlife is a time of depression, stress, frustration, crankiness, and all-around misery that calls for mood-altering drugs.

The most often reinforced myth in the media is that midlife is an inherently stressful time that women are not capable of handling without mood-altering drugs, sleep aids, and hormone therapy. The ad on television that I hate the most, the one that causes me to throw popcorn at the screen, is one where a middle-aged woman can't get a shopping cart unstuck from a rack of carts. The male voice-over informs her that she needs an antidepressant drug to help handle the stress of … the *shopping cart*! Well, he calls it something else but it is, after all, merely a shopping cart.

Have you ever had a tussle with a shopping cart? Of course! We all have. What did we do? We found… another cart! We don't need to medicate ourselves because of trauma over this, regardless of ads that try to make us believe we're too mentally incompetent to figure this out. That ad and many others are insulting to our intelligence.

Another concern about this kind of advertising is that it sends a message to people of all ages that midlife women are nincompoops. Have you seen an ad that you find insulting, one that portrays middle-aged women in an unflattering way? If so, don't ever buy that product.

The reality is that midlife doesn't have to be any more or less stressful than any other time of life. In fact, one research study found that if women expected the transition into midlife to be stressful, it was. If they didn't expect it to be stressful, it wasn't. Our expectations become self-fulfilling prophecies [13].

Another study found that 72.5 percent of 103 middle-aged women rated themselves as happy or very happy [8]. A three-year study of 541 midlife women concluded that the majority did not have negative consequences related to menopause [6]. In her book *If Not Now, When?* Stephanie Marston writes that the women she studied "experience midlife as a time of renewal and rebirth…one of the best times of their lives" [14]. Christiane Northrup, M.D., in *The Wisdom of Menopause*, says that "our midlife brains and bodies are set up to heal our past," allowing for contentment like we've never known [12]. The women in my study overwhelmingly indicated that midlife is a time for gaining perspective and delighting in all that life has to offer [15].

With a number of studies declaring that most midlife women are okay, which doesn't do drug companies any good, it's no wonder those companies spent $1.5 billion in 2001 to market their antidepressants to doctors, especially general practitioners, and $200 million on television and print ads aimed at customers. This could possibly explain why general practitioners, not psychiatrists, write the majority of antidepressant drug prescriptions [16]. Psychiatrists, by the very nature of their training and experience, are more likely to understand the need to face and deal with problems in order to expel them rather than shutting them into a closet of the brain and pretending they're not there, affording those problems the opportunity to leap out and scare you spitless at any moment.

One woman who had formerly been on an antidepressant for three years told me that the bugaboo is that drugs don't make your problems go away, they just make you not care about them. She said, "You either have to stay on drugs forever so you'll never care about your problems or you have to get off the drugs and learn to deal with your life."

Another woman revealed that she was in a drug haze for four years, precious years that are now lost to her. Her most vivid memories are of sleeping a lot.

Yet another woman who had a bad experience with antidepressants said she suspects the drug companies are in collusion with a bunch of "money mongers" who want to make sure that midlife women just shut up because we're a great big group who could have a lot of power. She said, "These guys want us to be quiet and let them continue to run things the same way they always have, to their advantage and not ours."

However, the antithesis of the experiences and contentions of those women is that of a woman who told of how she and her daughter had the appropriate medical testing done, ascertaining that they genuinely lack a chemical (serotonin) that is necessary to make the brain function properly. She believes that in their cases the deficiency is hereditary because many women in her family have suffered from the same symptoms, lethargy and depression. Prozac has dramatically changed her life and her daughter's life for the better. She says, "I'll do whatever it takes to stay on that stuff forever, and my husband will also make sure I do whatever it takes."

There is a small percentage of midlife women who are seriously depressed, often because of hormone or other chemical imbalances in their systems [17]. One survey found that about 9.5 percent of all Americans meet the criteria for mood disorder, but not all of them require medication [16]. Dr. Randy Martin, health correspondent for ABC News in Atlanta, reports that medical research indicates that about 5 percent of women genuinely need antidepressant drugs [18]. That means the other 95 percent of us do not.

Linda Hughes, Ed.D.

In my experience working with so many women, far more than 5 percent are on antidepressant drugs. There are too many women out there walking around in a drug-induced daze, inspiring Maureen Dowd of the New York Times to call this the "Zombie Nation" [19]. Why do so many women who don't need drugs take them? Some research indicates that depression can indeed be culturally manipulated by media messages that tell midlife women that they no longer fit the norm [13] and are supposed to be depressed as they age. The main problem, in that case, is that media messages depict women in negative and debilitating ways. Taking drugs won't change that. Our diligence in ignoring manipulative media messages and their products will.

What about you? Did you go to your doctor with normal symptoms of depression or stress and were you automatically put on a mood-altering drug without testing to see if you really need it? Sporadic, moderate depression and stress are normal parts of life. One TV ad says if you've been depressed for two weeks you need their drug. Please! If you've never been depressed for two weeks you're not living! Life has its ups and downs. You want the downs to get higher and the ups to get higher. You don't want to just get high.

Dowd says that ads make it seem like we all need drugs "for everything from shyness to smoking to work stress to supermom jits to severe premenstrual blues to muscle tension to dating anxiety" [19]. My personal favorite is "generalized stress anxiety." That fits everyone I know at some time or another. Arthur A. Levin, director of

22

the Center for Medical Consumers, said, "The symptomatology is so broad and vague that almost any one of us could say, yeah, that is me"[16]. Drug companies keep making up new names for disorders and new names for products because, as Dowd says, they are "addicted to their billion-dollar sales" [19].

But have you ever noticed some of the side effects of those pills? Feeling emotionally flat, sexual dysfunction, memory loss, insomnia, sleepiness, weight gain, weight loss, diarrhea... If you're not depressed before you take them you sure could be after.

Before you take any kind of drug, be it an antidepressant, a sleep aid, or hormone therapy, pay attention to your own body and mind, do your own homework, and consult a variety of trusted professional healthcare providers so that you can make a decision about taking a drug based upon information that applies to you, not based upon media hype. If the problem is biological, you might need medication. However, if the problem is that thing called *life*, other options are available, as you'll see in the chapters to come.

Midlife Myth #2:

Menopausal women are hot flashing enough energy to light up Las Vegas.

Remember pajama parties when you were a teenager? After eating copious amounts of junk food, listening to sappy records, dancing wildly, gossiping about boys, putting each others' hair up into French twists, and sticking someone's bra in the freezer, you'd settle down to tell scary stories. Until the suggestion was made that at night the Blob hid in *your* closet, out of millions of closets in the world, you'd never thought of it. But once the thought was planted in your head, it wouldn't go away. After that, you had to check every night before going to bed just to make sure the gooey monster hadn't slipped past you and squeezed into your tiny closet in order to roll out and smother you in your sleep.

Hot flashes are like that. In cultures where women don't expect to have them, they don't. In our culture, where there's lots of talk about them, many women fear them, fret about them, and end up having them. Even considering that in other cultures heredity, diet, and environment might have an affect on menopausal symptoms, it's interesting that in our culture those women who expect hot flashes get them and those who are thinking of other things don't [13].

That means that if you sit around waiting for the monster to get you, it will. If you're too busy doing other things, it won't.

The statistics about menopausal symptoms are so confusing that when I began researching midlife women, I took as many medical studies as I could find about hot flashes and looked at them all together. Findings ranged from 10 percent to 50 percent of menopausal women experiencing hot flashes. The consensus was that about 30 percent experience identifiable hot flashes and less than 20 percent have them severely enough to merit medical attention [15].

24

One woman I talked to made a good point. She said, "I think I might be having hot flashes, but I don't really know. I've noticed I feel more flushed and hotter when I work out. But maybe that's just because now I'm thinking about it and never did when I was younger. Maybe I've always been this flushed and hot when I work out."

Maybe you'll get hot flashes and maybe you won't. Maybe you already have them and want to make a concerted effort to divert your attention to other things. Maybe you're the one or two out of ten that needs medical attention. Whatever your situation, don't assume that hot flashes are a monstrous part of menopause that will attack you. Most midlife women are cool as a cucumber, some experience a warm glow, and only a few could light up Las Vegas.

Midlife Myth #3:

The moment a woman hits midlife she never wants to have sex again.

Ruby is fifty-three years old and says, "I know my body isn't like it used to be, but having a great body when I was younger didn't do me a damn bit of good 'cuz I was too stupid back then to enjoy sex the way it's meant to be." Like so many young women, she says she was worried about appearance, performance, and frequency. Now her only concern is doing what she and her husband want. "We don't try to keep up with what we see in movies. We don't care what anybody else is doing." A vibrant woman who lets her long gray hair hang lose, wears colorful flowing clothes, and makes no bones about loving to have sex, Ruby thinks that sexual intercourse is "good for the soul."

An added benefit for Ruby, one that is reported by a number of midlife women, was the fact that she no longer had to worry about getting pregnant after going through menopause. "It was the most wonderful thing in the world!" she exclaimed. "Harry and I have had more fun in the last three years than we had in twenty years before."

Are you surprised by Ruby's statements? Were you under the impression, as so many people are, that women in midlife are no longer interested in or not physically able to have sex?

Since ancient times women have known how to continue to have comfortable sexual intercourse after their bodies go through menopausal changes. Using creams for lubrication, midlife women have enjoyed coupling for as long as recorded history has been recording. Today, creams and other remedies take care of the drying of the vagina that occurs for most women as they age. It's no different than having dry skin. You put cream on that, too.

There are women, however, who don't want to continue to have sexual intercourse after menopause and that's a viable choice that needs to be respected in this rather sex-crazed culture in which we live. However, some of those women find that the desire for celibacy is temporary while they adjust to physical changes, which is something like learning to accept the physical changes of puberty that they recall from earlier in their lives.

Most women adjust to their physical changes and find that their sexuality develops in ways that delight rather than dismay them. Instead of *hormonal passion* like they had when they were younger, they now have *intentional passion*.

A woman named Jessie put it this way: "When we were young, we'd just look at each other and had to have sex. We didn't think about it, we just did it. Now we think about it – sometimes for days or weeks before we do it. We flirt outrageously, knowing we don't have to fall on our knees and have sex that very moment. It's so much fun! It's a new kind of sex, where there's an emotional connection and physical. It's the best sex in the world!"

Women have said things like, "I used to be too self-conscious to play games, like being the French maid, but I'm not anymore, as long as he'll be Superman once in awhile," "Variety is good, like in new places," and "I love it that as we've matured my husband and I understand each other's needs so much better than we used to." One thing about sex that comes up over and over is fun. Midlife women feel freer than they did when they were younger.

Because ego is no longer tied up in sexuality, midlife women are free to have fun! Instead of being hurt if her husband says, "Not while the game is on," she knows that his disinterest is most likely temporary and is not a comment on his feelings for her. It doesn't mean, "I don't love you." It means, "I'd really like to watch this game. Let's do the sex thing later." By midlife we've learned the difference.

What if a man does lose interest in having sex with a woman he's been with for many years? If the woman has matured sexually, able to let go and enjoy sex without insecurities and constraints, most men, barring a medical condition, will not lose interest. Let's face it. They like to have sex. They put fewer constraints on it than we do. Many midlife couples who have been together throughout their entire young adulthood enjoy sex together until their bodies become decrepit and just stop responding. You don't have to worry about that for a long time.

But what if a woman loses interest? Women fear that *hormonal* passion will die as they age. It does. Sexual desire can wane. Thankfully, however, it's replaced by a better kind of *intentional* passion where we know what we're doing. That causes most women, even those who lost interest in sex while going through menopause, to discover a renewed interest in their sexuality.

We don't worry anymore about measuring up to movie star standards like whether our thighs are too big or our breasts are too small. We don't worry about whether we're having sex often enough to keep up with the national average. We don't even worry about our wrinkles and flaws, knowing that it's likely our partner's eyesight isn't any better than ours and they can't see those little things anyway. Our only concern is sharing one of life's ultimate pleasures with someone for whom we feel a sense of communion, a sense of genuine sharing.

Besides, the reality is that a majority of married women will be widowed when they become elderly. That means the opportunity to have sexual intercourse won't be available forever, so we might as well enjoy it while we can.

More Myths

There are even more myths about midlife, like the beliefs that at age 40 the body goes to hell and never comes back, that the middle-aged mind not only wanders it leaves altogether, that women are traumatized by the "empty nest syndrome," that women go through "stages" of midlife, that midlife women don't have the skills necessary in today's job market, and that we no longer like to have fun. The following chapters dispel those myths, too, so keep going.

Create Your Own Myths

1. Are there family stories about midlife that you've heard forever, stories that you assume to be true? For example, "Menopause is just awful for all of the women in this family. A hysterectomy is the only way to go." Or, "Aunt Lucinda says that drugs saved her during the change, so they'll save you, too." Write down stories you've heard for so long they've become unconscious ways of thinking.

_____

_____

_____

_____

   Is this the way you want to think or would you like to change your personal story? What do you want your own story to be?

_____

_____

_____

_____

_____

_____

2. Are there societal stories about midlife that you've heard forever, stories that you assume to be true? For example, "Men always leave older women for younger women." The

myths in this chapter are examples of those types of urban myths. Write down some other ones you've heard.

_____

_____

_____

_____

_____

3. Do you want to think that way just because everybody else does or would you rather create your own story? How will your story be different?

_____

_____

_____

_____

_____

4. Look at your LifeMap on page 15 and ask yourself if the stories, the myths, that you carry around in your head are stopping you from creating the LifeMap that you want. Dan P. McAdams, Ph.D., in his book *The Stories We Live By: Personal Myths and the Making of the Self,* says, "A personal myth is an act of imagination that is a patterned integration of our remembered past, perceived present, and anticipated future... We do not discover ourselves in myth; we *make*

ourselves through myth" [20]. If you are going to make yourself through your own myths, what do you want those myths to be? What do *you* want to be?

_____

_____

_____

_____

_____

_____

5.   Consider how you can incorporate your own personal myths into your life. Keep these ideas in mind as you work with your LifeMap.

Chapter 3 ~ The Center of Your LifeMap: Your Soul

"The soul, like the moon, is new, and always new again."
Lalleswari, 14th Century

When I asked women to describe their souls, responses included:

"My soul is the center of my being, the point at which I know that my life is my own."

"Soul is what you instinctively know to be right, deep down inside."

"That's a tough one, but I think it's my inner self."

"I'm too busy to think about that."

"Huh?"

When was the last time you thought about your soul? You might talk about soul in church and hear about it in songs, but have you genuinely thought about what it means to you?

I like what Thomas Moore says in his book *Care of the Soul:*

It is impossible to define precisely what the soul is.
Definition is an intellectual enterprise anyway; the soul
prefers to imagine. We know intuitively that soul has
to do with genuineness and depth, as when we say

Linda Hughes, Ed.D.

certain music has soul or a remarkable person is
soulful.... Soul is revealed in attachment, love, and
community, as well as in retreat on behalf of inner
communing... [21]

Moore is saying that soul has to do with connecting with
others as well as with connecting with oneself. We usually think of a
person who is seeking her soul as trekking up a mountain to meditate
in solitary bliss in order to open her being to divine revelations. That's
one way of connecting to your soul. But another way that you will get
to know your "power of character," as James Hillman describes soul
in *The Soul's Code [22]*, is to connect to other people and to pay
attention to what you're doing while you do it.

What's a Soul?

The medieval word "hal" is the root of modern words like
hale, hearty, healthy, whole, and holy [23]. That's an amazing list of
words that are all connected to one another, words that aptly describe
what it's like to feel connected to your soul. When your soul system is
in balance, with intentional links to the other areas of your life, you
feel hale, hearty, healthy, and whole. As a result, the experience of
daily living becomes holy.

Making connections amongst the disparate areas of your life
and allowing for balanced living are what it takes to know your own
soul. But there are as many ways to connect to one's soul as there are
human beings on earth. We each have our own way of thinking about

our souls, if we give them any thought at all, and our own ways of feeling as though we're honoring them.

Sally, a minister, says that she feels most connected to her soul early in the morning when she arises before anyone else is up in her house. She has a cup of coffee by herself, sipping it slowly while looking out the window. "That's my time of day," she says. "The time when my thoughts are my own. Sometimes I mull over important things and sometimes I couldn't tell you later what I was thinking about. I just do whatever I need to do. Then everybody gets up and my attention turns to them." Sally perhaps epitomizes Moore's description of soul as being community with others as well as inner communing. It's the balance between the two that makes Sally feel whole.

Betty, an office manager, explains that she feels closest to her inner self, her soul, when she's outdoors. "I just have to be outside," she declares. "If I don't get outside for a long period of time, like if the weather is bad or I'm sick, I feel like my world is all lop-sided. I have to see some trees in order to feel sane."

Wendy, a midlife student, has another way of thinking about her soul. "My body is my soul and my soul is my body. They're one and the same. Yoga is the best way in the world to get in touch with your body/soul."

Teresa, a homemaker, told me that she's acutely aware of "this thing called a soul" every time she looks into her little girl's eyes. "You can see it. Whatever it is, it's there. And it's so beautiful!"

35

Kate, a Native American elementary school teacher, believes that all living things have souls – people, animals, and plants. "My people don't think of the soul as something separate like white people do. It's what we are. It is us. It's each of us alone and all of us together. It's us in connection with the earth and the sky. There's no such thing as a soul out there all by itself."

Rose, a psychic healer, explains that your soul is not something that is inside of you. Everything that you are or ever could be is inside of your soul. She says, "Your soul encompasses everything, nurtures and protects everything else that you are and say and do and feel and think. That's why it's so important to acknowledge and respect and take care of your soul."

Virginia, a corporate executive, likes the physical work and camaraderie that comes from helping build Habitat for Humanity houses. "There's nothing better," she contends. "You work hard and become friends while building a house. When you're done you feel like you've really accomplished something. That's when I feel closest to God. That's when I know I was put here on earth to share with others."

Anna Marie, a writer, declares that the best way to get in touch with your soul is to honor the movement of the earth and the seasons. On the eve of each month's full moon, she goes into her backyard and stands in the center of a circle of stones that she has made, looks up at the moon, and prays to the Holy Spirit. "I thank the Holy One for this life and pray for peace in the world," she says. "If it rains," she notes,

"I sit inside and have a nice glass of wine. That works pretty well, too."

Personally, I like to pray each morning at a window in my bedroom that looks out over our backyard. Our puppy, Mandy, usually sits beside me and it's amazing that this hyperactive little creature seems to instinctively know this is a special time. She lies still and waits for me to finish. Sometimes I read from prayer books, sometimes I make it up as I go along, and sometimes just I lie in the sun and gaze out. As often as the weather permits I open the window. I might light a scented candle. I pray for what's happening in my life and for what's happening in the world. I always thank the Holy Spirit and my guides for being there for me. On days when I have to leave home early and skip prayer time, the day never seems to go as well. When I begin my day with that time just for me and the wonders of life, the world seems like a better place to be in because I'm in a better place within myself. I'm in tune with my soul.

As you were just reading through other women's ways and my way of connecting with our souls, you might have found yourself saying, "Yeah, I do that, too" or "I'd like to do that." You might have run into some where you thought, "No, not for me." That's good. It helps you get ideas about what you might be doing that works for you or what you want to start doing that will lead you to your soul.

Getting to Know Your Soul

1. What did you just read about that you do, too, that makes you feel balanced and whole, like you are in connection with your soul?

   _____

2. Was there nothing there that's similar to what you do? What do you do?

   _____

   _____

3. Is there something, either that you read about here or that you know about on your own, that you would like to start to do in order to honor your soul?

   _____

   _____

4. When will you begin?

   _____

Chapter 4 ~ Your Body

"I've got a stomach now as well as a behind.
And I mean – well, you can't pull it in both ways, can you?
I've made it a rule to pull in my stomach and let my behind look after
itself."
Agatha Christie, 1960

People say that all children are beautiful, but whenever my sister and I want a good laugh we get out old photos of me when I was two years old. I look like a miniature sumo wrestler that someone tried to make look like a little girl by curling her hair and dressing her in ruffles. I was not a pretty child, although my mother always insisted, as only a mother can, that I was.

Even though there had never been any indication whatsoever that this would happen, when I was a teen I still held delusions that someday I'd grow up to look like my tall, slender, gorgeous mom and her sisters. So clearly I remember a day when I was fifteen watching one of my cousins, who had inherited the model-like family female build, walk across a room at school. I thought, "She's so beautiful and graceful – she looks like a swan." Then reality struck like a sledgehammer. "And I'm a duck!" It had been three years since I'd grown taller. I was 5'3" and was going to stay that way. My legs were always going to be short. I'd never "slimmed down" much and probably wouldn't without a lot of work. I didn't even have their lush, thick hair.

As dismaying as that was when I was a teen, as I've aged I've wondered if it's harder for beautiful women who age, if they feel more like they've "lost" something when their looks change. For many of us, we didn't have that much to "lose," so aging is just a continuation of working with what we've got like we've always done. There's an old Hollywood story that many years ago Helen Hayes and Ruth Gordon, better known as character actors than as glamorous movie stars, were in the studio commissary when a couple of famous actresses walked in. All eyes turned to the beauties. Ruth said to Helen, "That's okay. After their looks have faded, we'll still be fun and interesting."

By the time I was in my twenties, I knew I'd better work on things other than beauty, like being fun, interesting, and healthy. In other words, I decided that if I was going to be a duck than I'd learn to swim as best I could. I started working out with weights, eating more healthily, and exercising. Since I wasn't going to be pretty in the traditional sense anyway, my goal always was to be healthy. And that's the only goal in terms of our bodies that makes any sense, especially as we age.

We all know that. So, why is it that so many midlife women agonize over their changing physiques, run to plastic surgeons, and torture themselves trying to recapture what they once were rather than enjoying what they are now? It could be because we've been inundated with messages for so long about how we're "supposed" to look that we lose sight of what's real and what isn't.

Barbie Bodies

In a study about the effect of magazines on college women, two groups of women were pre-tested to ascertain what they considered to be society's ideal body type. No difference was found between the two groups. Then one group viewed women's fashion magazines while the other group looked at news magazines. After just 13 minutes, women viewing fashion magazines thought than an ideal body weight was lower than the women who looked at news magazines. Just a few minutes of looking at fashion magazine images changed their minds about what is a perfect weight for a woman! [24]

It's no wonder that after 30 years of looking at magazines and other media messages midlife women have a difficult time separating fact from fiction. For example, cultural studies researcher Linda Wolszon states:

> The ideal for the female body, represented by actresses, models, and Miss America contestants, represents the thinnest 5 percent of women…. The fact that 95% of women cannot measure up to this ideal…is thought to be a central reason why a majority of women surveyed report significant dissatisfaction with their current body size and shape—a dissatisfaction

that has been empirically linked to lower self-esteem,

[and] depression.... [25]

So, of course, a fifty-year-old woman could feel that she doesn't "measure up," especially if she's been comparing herself to unrealistic standards since her teens. It's easy to see how some women, after years of being told they are supposed to be thin, young, and attractive, could become depressed about their changing looks.

Yes, Attitude is Everything

How do you feel about your changing looks? One study found an important factor in a woman's ability to adjust to her midlife physique: How you think about your body is as important as the actual changes your body is going through. If you accept yourself you are more likely to be happy. If you don't accept yourself you are more likely to be unhappy. The actual physical changes are the same in either case [13].

Another study indicates that there is a gap between what actually happens to a woman's body as she ages and what she thinks has happened, with women viewing their bodies as exhibiting more change, for example percent of weight gain, than has actually occurred [26]. Those studies tell us that we need to give ourselves a break and stop trying to be like women in ads, on TV, or in the movies.

Unfortunately, lots of women don't give themselves a break and consider their overweight bodies to be their greatest failures in life [27]. In her wonderful book, *If Not Now, When?* Stephanie Marston says she believes that rejection of one's own aging body is a type of self-hatred that is constructed out of fear. She quotes Judith Viorst as saying:

> For if youth is linked to beauty, and beauty is linked to a woman's sexual attractiveness, and her sexual attractiveness is important to her winning and holding a man, then age's assaults on beauty can catapult her into a terror of abandonment. [14]

Yet it's seems that women are more critical of their bodies than men are. You might have seen some of the magazine articles over the years that report that wives consistently rate their own bodies as less attractive than their husbands do. It's possible that when a woman is worried about "holding" a man, her worries and negative attitude about her body affect the relationship more than her body shape.

Your attitude about your body plays a key role in your ability to be happy. A woman who sees herself as a failure because she doesn't measure up to the media's ideal body type is not going to be happy in midlife and beyond. Conversely, a woman who defines the ideal body for herself and doesn't worry about external messages is going to be more open to all of the changes, physical and otherwise, that will ensue in her middle years. A midlife woman has the incredible opportunity, after years of trying to fit someone else's mold, to create her own measure for physical beauty, and the best measure for that is health.

Getting Along with Yer Giddyup and Other Helpful Hints

There are two pet peeves of mine that I often see when I'm in groups of women: 1) Some women wear their clothes so tight, especially their slacks, that they advertise their giddyups and everything else they've got to the world and, 2) some women wear dumb shoes. Not only do these things look bad, they are unhealthy for the body.

Pants that pull in the crotch are pants that are too tight. They contribute to urinary tract and vaginal infections that women are too prone to anyway. Tight clothes chafe, transmit dampness and bacteria, cut off circulation, and imprison one's poor skin. Women need to buy clothes in the size that they are, not the size they used to be or wish they were. The body needs to be able to breathe and move comfortably. As one woman said, "I've quit wearing control-top pantyhose because I finally figured out that they're not made for human beings."

Now, if you think I'm saying women shouldn't dress nicely, you're mistaken. Women can dress very nicely and still be kind to their bodies. In my seminars I sometimes ask, "Who is at this very moment wearing something that's uncomfortable?" About a quarter of the women are honest and raise their hands. Then I ask, "Who is totally comfortable and you know you look good, too?" A number of women will raise their hands and the more gregarious will model their

44

clothes for us. And they do look good. Best of all, while looking at them the observer's mind doesn't wander off to prickly thoughts like "Ouch…those pants hurt just to look at" or "Owww…her feet must be killing her in those shoes!" Think about it. You notice those things on other women, which means they notice those things about you. Edith Head, the famous movie costume designer from the '30s & '40s, is reported to have once said that a woman's clothes should be tight enough to show that she's a woman but lose enough to show that she's a lady.

Shoes are another health hazard for women, especially what Oprah calls "ten-minute shoes," the ones you can only stand to have on your feet for ten minutes. They might look interesting but they're not made for walking. Medical research indicates that years of wearing high-heels causes debilitating problems later in life for many women. The feet become deformed and need surgery. The back sways and knees become arthritic. The derriere protrudes an extra 25 percent. (Some of us don't need any extra in that region.) And the foot has a hard time readjusting to lower heeled shoes. It's recommended that if you've worn high heels for a long time that you start buying lower heels in ½ inch increments until you get to 1 ½ inches, which is the highest heel any of us should be wearing [28, 29].

My husband has heard me talk about this so much that one day when we were in a mall walking behind a woman in a very short skirt and very high heels, he said, "I used to think shoes like that were sexy. But now that I know how damaging they are to a woman's body, they just look ignorant." (He didn't comment on the skirt.)

Midlife women shudder at the thought of starting to wear "more sensible" clothes. But I'm here to tell you that you can be sensible, stylish, and healthy all at the same time. As Gilda Radner once said on *Saturday Night Live*, "I base my fashion taste on what doesn't itch." Good advice. Don't wear anything that itches or hitches.

Swans and Ducks Unite for Health

One of the midlife myths is that after age forty the body goes to hell and never comes back. Get healthy and your body will not go to hell. Even if it was on its way, you can redeem it. Don't let yourself get away with the excuse, "It's too late." Unless you're dead, it's never too late.

Whether you were born a swan or a duck, it's never too late to learn to swim and stay afloat for a long, healthy life. Eat well, exercise at least moderately, don't smoke, don't wear *anything* that hurts, and change your attitude if you need to. Changing your mind about your body will help you take better care of yourself. It'll help you understand that you don't "have" a body, your body is an integrated part of your soul and, like every other facet of your being, needs your acceptance, love, and care.

Your Body and Your LifeMap

1. Look back at your LifeMap on page 15 and think about the line or absence of a line drawn between your Soul and your Body.

2. If there is a connection, are you happy with that connection? ____ If so, what can you do to continue to strengthen the connection? _____ If there is a connection but you're not happy with it, what can you do to begin to strengthen that connection?

   _____

3. If there is no connection between your Soul and your Body, what can you do *now* to begin to build a connection? (e.g. Hike, workout, dance, bike ride, walk your dog, swing, practice yoga, stretch, meditate, lift weights, exercise to workout videos, join a healthy eating program, stop drinking soda, stop drinking alcohol, drink more water, stop smoking, wear more comfortable clothes, stop wearing stupid shoes, roll down a hill like you did when you were a kid, swim, ski, dig in the dirt….well, you get the idea.)

   _____

   _____

   _____

4. Which one are you going to do *today*?

   _____

5. Take off your clothes and look at yourself in a mirror. (This is recommended when alone at home!) I know you don't want to. As

one woman said, "If God wanted me naked he would have made my skin fit better." But do it anyway. Take a long, unemotional look. This is you. Whether or not you like what you see, be thankful you have this body because without it you would not have life.

6. Remember that this is your own unique body. How other people look, like women in magazines or on TV, have absolutely nothing to do with *your* body. They have no control over *your* body. Only you can do that. Looking like someone else is not your goal. Looking like a healthy you is your goal.

7. Make a promise to yourself that you will take care of your body, that you will do the healthy things you just listed. You will nurture your body and listen to what it tells you. You will not ignore it, as you've probably done in the past. You will respect it for the life that it gives you.

8. Write a prayer or meditation, even one sentence, which you can say daily to thank the Holy Spirit for your body of life. Then repeat it every day of your life.

_____

_____

_____

Chapter 5 ~ Your Mind

"It is all right to say exactly what you think if you have learned to think exactly."

Marcelene Cox, 1945

There's the old saying that sometimes your mind doesn't wander, it leaves altogether. Then there's the one about "old-timer's" disease. And the notion that a woman can never make up her mind.

If you've been depending on these types of excuses to cover your mistakes and forgetfulness, forget it. Those alibis don't fly. If you're in midlife, you're not going to start having memory variations until much later in life. Even then you aren't likely to forget things; you'll just take longer to retrieve information [30].

It works like this: When you're young you park your car at the mall, stay inside for four hours, and come out to walk straight to your car. In later life you park your car at the mall, stay inside for twenty minutes, and come out to stand at the entrance, trying to remember where you parked. You will remember, it'll just take a couple of minutes to pull that information up from the brain file it's been stored in. It's not until you're much older, in your eighties or nineties that you might forget where you are and will look for the car you owned twenty years earlier. And, you might not be forgetful at all, beating a path to your vehicle.

Linda Hughes, Ed.D.

So, you might be wondering what is going on when you do forget things. It's frustrating losing your keys, missing an important meeting, or totally blanking out on your mother's name when you go to introduce her at a party. You need not fear. You've always been like that! Most people have memory lapses all of their lives. We just don't worry about them when we're younger. We don't start to fret until we begin to fall for the myths of midlife, believing that we will now become debilitated. Poppycock! But if you're concerned, anyway, here are some things you can do to keep your mind sharp as a little tack.

Feed Your Brain

Just like you take care of the rest of your body, you can take care of your brain. Some things are no-brainers: get enough sleep, eat right, and exercise. Another way to nourish your brain is to learn. Let yourself absorb new information for the rest of your life, granting yourself life-long learning. It's one of the best ways to keep those little brain synapses sharp, open your mind to new possibilities, and make life interesting.

In case you haven't officially attended school for a long time and question whether you're capable of learning at this age, you are. No doubt about it. You might need to dust that gray matter off a little, but it's able to gather and assess information until the day you get your toe tag.

Sometimes women are concerned about IQ tests they took years ago, ones that said they weren't as smart as they thought they were or wanted to be. Did you know that those old IQ tests are now considered to be so limited in scope that the findings are virtually useless? Of course, this is bad news if you came up a genius back then; but, don't worry, you might still be one today. If you're not a genius, you're at least smart. (You were intelligent enough to pick up this book, weren't you?)

Howard Gardner is an educator who's done a lot of research on what he calls "Multiple Intelligences" [31]. He believes there are many different ways that a person can be smart, but most of those ways are not recognized and appreciated as much as they should be. He lists eight categories of intelligence: (1) linguistic, (2) logical-mathematical, (3) musical, (4) spatial, (5) bodily kinesthetic, (6) intrapersonal, (7) interpersonal, and (8) natural. Most IQ tests only measure the first two, ignoring all of the others. Musical ability could be playing an instrument, singing, or writing music. Spatial means an ability to visualize objects in context in space, like an architect would do. An example of someone with bodily kinesthetic ability is a high diver, a person who is in tune with her physicality and knows how to use it. Intrapersonal is a sort of inner wisdom; interpersonal is skill at connecting and dealing with others; and, natural is one who feels at home in nature, with spiritual connotations.

Do you see yourself in any of those categories? Do you have abilities that aren't measured on tests? Forget about tests you took when you were a kid. Give yourself credit for what you are capable of

51

doing now. Are there abilities that you'd like to develop? Remember it all begins in your mind. If you think that you can't do it, you won't. If you think that you can, you will.

How Women Learn

Anthropologist Mary Catherine Bateson, daughter of the famous anthropologist Margaret Meade, describes a woman's life as being like a quilt, with a variety of patchwork pieces that can't be appreciated until viewed as a whole. If a single piece, a single aspect of the woman's life, is analyzed, "The pattern and loving labor in the patchwork is lost" [32]. We live, work, play, love, and learn within the context of our worlds. We don't separate our emotions from our thoughts; we don't see ourselves as islands without connection to others; and, we don't think that we should. At times we've pieced together life patches that were misfits, so we used them as reference points for piecing together better lives. If you haven't done that yet, you can.

Learning from the past by reflecting on it helps us know what we need to do in the present. Reflecting, however, is different from what a lot of people do. They ruminate, becoming stuck in what happened way back when, reliving it by retelling it (at least to themselves) time and again, and allowing themselves to feel like victims. Reflecting means that you look at that piece of your life and say, "I don't ever want to do that again. What can I learn from that to

52

make sure I don't repeat it?" Rumination keeps you immobilized. Reflection moves you forward.

In order to figure out what else to do, as women we first must come to value our best ways of learning, which have not traditionally been revered in our culture. You might not have time to go pick up a college degree, which is valued as a valid form of knowledge collection, but you do have the ability to learn informally and incidentally. To do that, you need to become aware of what you're doing.

Informal learning is that which you do "on the side." You take a yoga class, attend a work seminar, and read a self-help book. Incidental learning is that which you don't plan at all, it just pops up. You're flipping through the TV channels and a show on forensic science comes on, and you plop down to watch the whole thing.

Informal and incidental learning are the ways that most of us gather our knowledge. Therefore, we want to be more conscious about what we select to pay attention to. Carefully choose the classes and seminars you attend. Be aware of what you watch on TV. When I surveyed 350 midlife women about watching television, the vast majority said that they don't watch much TV. Then when I asked what they do watch, those same women would list their ten favorite shows. (*JAG* was the #1 favorite.) They didn't think they watched much television, but because it's on in the background in most homes, they were watching much more than they realized. We want to be aware of what we're doing and spend our learning time well. We learn in social context, in the middle of all that is going on around us. That means we're exposed to a lot of good stuff and a lot of junk.

You can pick out the strong, functional parcels of learning that will enhance your quilt of life and toss out the tattered rags. Remember that just because something is said by a friend, a stranger, or in the media, that doesn't mean it fits for you. You decide what does.

A Word from the Wise

That would be you – the wise one. One of the truly spectacular things about aging is the wisdom we acquire along the way. We really do get smarter. We stop making the same mistakes over-and-over. We stop beating ourselves up over every little thing we've ever done wrong. We even stop thinking of ourselves as being "wrong."

Time and again when I talk to women they say they wouldn't trade the wisdom of age for anything they had in youth. They say things like, "Uh-uh. You couldn't make me be twenty again and be as much of a lunkhead as I was back then," "I wouldn't trade the peace of being wiser for anything," and "Thank goodness I stopped marrying men like my second husband. Who knows what my brain was doing – obviously nothing – when I married him!" Dorothy Parker once said that every woman should have a middle husband that she can forget, and some of us have had them. We wouldn't go back to that kind of melee for all the diamonds in Elizabeth Taylor's vault.

Many midlife women find that they're smarter in many areas of their lives – relationships, finance, work, personal care – then ever before.

Wisdom carries with it a kind of practicality and sagacity that simply were not possible in our youth. It takes time to learn to navigate life's tidal waves and lulls. We've opened our minds and no longer see things as black or white, instead seeing a colorful multitude of possibilities. As educators Sharan Merriam and Rosemary Caffarella remind us, "Wisdom involves special types of experience-based knowledge and is characterized by the ability to move away from absolute truth, to be reflective, and to make sound judgments related to everyday life" [30].

If you're wondering whether or not you have wisdom, chances are you do, you're just not accustomed to listening to yourself when you give yourself a word from the wise. Do you often reprimand yourself for not following your instincts? Do you feel like you have inner wisdom and good intuition, but don't follow them? Do you find yourself saying, "I knew I shouldn't do that!" Well, why did you do it? You knew better. Listen to yourself when you tell yourself what you need to know.

Ha! Ha!

Along with wisdom comes the knowledge that not everything in life is a do or die situation. Humor pokes through the shell of seriousness that envelopes too many people and we finally relax so that we can enjoy life. Not that we don't understand the importance of

Linda Hughes, Ed.D.

our existences. We do. We just don't see any reason to be grim about it.

Psychologist Joan Erikson wrote, "The world being full of incongruities, perplexity would surely be overwhelming if humor abandoned us.... When we can even see ourselves as funny, it eases this daily living in such close proximity with ourselves" [30]. Laughing at ourselves, not in derision but in joy, is one of the great treasures of aging.

If you don't have many opportunities to laugh, find some. You might not like comediennes who are raunchy, or you might, but there are also those who have "clean" routines. Find the type of laugher that tickles all of your bones and allow yourself time to enjoy it. Go to a comedy club or watch comedy routines on television. Listen to your seven-year-old grandchild's silly jokes. (The one I heard today was, "Why did the robber take a bath? So he could make a clean getaway.") Watch *Everybody Loves Raymond* on TV. Go to a fun movie. Make up your own jokes. As Jessamyn West suggested, "A good time for laughing is when you can" [33].

It's Your Mind – Do What You Wanna Do

In midlife you don't have to live according to the constraints of what you parents told you when you were a child, of what you learned when you attended school, or of what others such as friends and the media have been telling you all of your life. You're a grown woman. You can make up your own mind and think for yourself. You can learn and laugh, reflect and cry, and experience hope and happiness like you never have before. Others may have claimed your mind in the past, but now it belongs to you. Embrace it, nurture it, and hear what it tells you about you.

Your Mind and Your LifeMap

1. Look back at your LifeMap on page 15 and think about the line or absence of a line drawn between your Soul and your Mind.

2. If there is a connection, are you happy with that connection? ____ If so, what can you do to continue to strengthen the connection?

   _____

3. If there is a connection but you're not happy with it, what can you do to begin to strengthen that connection?

   _____

4. If there is no connection between your Soul and your Mind, what can you do *now* to begin to build a connection? (E.g. Take continuing education classes that are offered by local schools, read books, watch educational television, join a discussion group like a book club, go back to college, talk to someone with different points of view from yours, look up information on the Internet, take a "distance learning" class on the Internet, listen to educational audiotapes, attend seminars, read newspapers and news magazines, and do cross-word puzzles. The possibilities are endless!)

   _____

   _____

   _____

5. Which one are you going to do *today?*

    _____

6. Review the Multiple Intelligences described in this chapter. Is there one you'd like to develop? _____ Which one? _____

7. What can you do to develop it?

    _____

8. Are you aware of your own "informal" and "incidental" learning?

    _____

9. What can you do to be more selective about how you learn and what you learn? (E.g. Be more careful about what you watch on television; read books for yourself rather than taking someone else's word about what they say; or select classes that will help you grow intellectually.)

    _____

    _____

    _____

10. Do you know a person whom you consider to be wise?

    _____

11. Who?

    _____

12. Do you have a chance to listen to that person tell her/his life stories?

    _____

13. If so, ask them to share with you. You might be delighted at what you learn about them and about yourself.

14. Do you have enough laughter in your life? _____ If not, where and with whom can you expose your self to more joy?

_____

Chapter 6 ~ Your Relationships

"The long-term accommodation that protects marriage and other such relationships is… forgetfulness."
Alice Walker, 1981

We all know that relationships can be thorny. We also know that they can be the best thing in life. As we age our relationships age, too, becoming more mature, more meaningful, and more fun than ever before. Some people believe that women are more relationship-oriented than men and aren't as concerned with acquiring power in the traditional sense, like in business, as with making connections throughout our lives [9].

In our culture, women are taught that we are the ones who are supposed to be nurturing and care about others. Men are taught that they are supposed to "succeed." In fact, when I studied women and the media I found that these portrayals were alarmingly prevalent in the movies and on TV [15]. I think that means that men are taught to live with a disadvantage. They might succeed in business but they don't do as well as women at being human beings who relate to others. Women, therefore, are the ones who "succeed" in the end because we attend to what matters in life - love.

Wouldn't it be grand if it weren't a matter of gender, one being more attuned to love than the other, but a matter of everyone appreciating the possibility that the primary purpose we're here on earth is to connect with and love others? Wouldn't it be a different world if we all did just that?

We may not be able to change the world, a fact which frustrates many women, but we can change our own little corners of it. If we each do that, eventually all of those corners will come together, like a huge universal quilt, and we will live in a better world. That might sound naïve, but what have we got to lose by giving it a try? Only heartache.

So, let's say that you want to bring as much love into your corner of the world as possible. Where do you begin? Connecting with your own soul is a good place to start. And one way that you can do that is by connecting with others.

Here Comes the Bride

Some women feel like they're failures if they're not married. Some who've had bad marriages and are divorced wouldn't walk down the aisle again if they were being stabbed with a cattle prod. And some think that marriage is a good thing if the relationship is good. Otherwise, it's not worth it. Marriage can be energizing if the relationship is healthy. That doesn't mean it won't have its hiccups, but it needs to be robust most of the time. If it's not a mutually respectful, satisfying situation, it's better to be single. There's no shame in expecting to be treated well. You deserve it.

Yet many women don't feel that they deserve good things. One woman I interviewed had a wonderful marriage, but when her husband succeeded in business beyond their wildest dreams and provided them with a luxurious home, she confided that she felt like she was "visiting" because that kind of nice place wasn't for little ole her. She'd been raised dirt poor. They spent their early married years in poverty and their middle years in moderate comfort. The leap to wealth was one that she'd never considered and had not yet made. I encouraged her to stretch her legs and make the jump. She and her husband had worked hard for many years and deserved everything that they had. The last time I talked to her she was doing much better, having just decorated with all new furniture. She was even considering buying a Harley for fun.

That example can be translated into relationships. Do you feel like you deserve good treatment from others? Do you let yourself have good relationships or are you stuck in "poverty" relationship thinking?

One of the surprising things I discovered about midlife women is that many who have difficult marriages do not want to toss out their husbands. Of course, there are wives who do want to heave ho spouses who are genuine jerks. But apart from real abuse, many women come to see their husbands as being not quite so jerky after all. Those women are over their adolescent fantasies of envisioning marriage like a kiss-the-frog-and-turn-him-into-a-prince movie, instead acccpting the reality that, like their husbands, they are a little froggy themselves sometimes.

Interestingly, some feel like they are in better positions than ever before to work on their marriages and heal them. This is the time of their lives when they feel strong, emotionally and spiritually, and therefore have the will to work on difficult issues.

They also, however, don't see so many things as being difficult. Husbands' behaviors and habits that might have bothered them when they were younger don't seem like such a big deal anymore. A woman told me about her husband's lax discipline of their children, which used to drive her crazy. Now that the kids were grown and gone, she said, "There's nothing about him that bugs me. I really like him a lot. And I know he'll spoil the grandkids, but somehow that doesn't bother me because for once in my life I'd like to relax and do a little spoiling, too."

Over time, whether it's a first, second, or higher-digit marriage, many couples seem to glide into a rhythm of being together. One woman even collects frog paraphernalia in honor of her husband. As Robert Fulghum put it in his book, *It Was on Fire When I Lay Down on It*, "They know that companionship in the kitchen around suppertime … and good company and friendship count for more than good looks. And they know that marrying a frog is fine if you really like the frog a whole lot and don't expect princely transformations…. The love tends to be richer, deeper, wiser …" [34].

Then Come the Children

Tearfully, a woman I'll call Kathleen recited the story of her nineteen-year-old son's most recent visit home from the Marines. He only had a couple of days off, so she was stunned when he told her that he was spending his nights in a hotel with his girlfriend instead of in his old bedroom at home. Kathleen sobbed, "I can't believe he wanted to stay with *her* instead of here with his family."

Out of a dozen women I interviewed on the topic, she was the only one in the throes of experiencing "empty nest syndrome." One other said she had felt it when her daughter first left for college, but "got over it within a couple of weeks." All of the others were quite happy when their chickadees spread their wings and flew the coop. A few were even, well, thrilled.

Women who feel depressed when their children leave are those who question their mothering abilities. According to counselor Laurel Lippert, a woman's inability to adjust to the change might indicate other issues "such as unresolved losses or poor coping skills" [6]. Not that mothers don't miss their offspring – they do. But most mothers are ready. After all, they have been anticipating and preparing for this transition for eighteen or more years. (Sometimes a lot more!) Mothers who feel confident in their parenting are proud to see their children go out and tackle the world on their own.

It's like teaching your child to ride a bike when she was little. At first you held on to the back bumper so she wouldn't fall.

Although your support pleased her at first, eventually it started to annoy her. She began to shout, "Let go! I can do it!" You were afraid she might veer off, hit a tree, or tumble into the street. But you finally let go. And whatever her course, it was her own. That was one of the most unselfish gifts you ever gave her.

In our middle years, it's time to let go of our grown children, time to let them live their own lives, making their own mistakes and garnering credit for their own successes. Amazingly, when we let go is when they are most likely to seek our company. Although they will always be our children, our relationships take on a new adult dimension that wasn't possible before.

Think back to the example of your solar system, rotating and expanding to include more space and more possibilities. When you do let go of your children, it's a whole new universe, one that is bigger than you ever imaged. Most of our kids don't get lost in space. Most return to visit our worlds, even bringing their alien spouses with them. If we're lucky, we find the aliens to be interesting and learn to love them, too. They turn out to be part of the expansion of our universes, part of our ability to bring more love into existence.

Parents

Sometimes Baby Boomers are called the "Sandwich Generation" because so many end up taking care of their children and their parents at the same time. We're in the middle, between those two generations. Whether your parents are independent or depend on you for their care, your relationship with them will last the rest of your life. Even if they, as they most likely will, die before you, your connection to them will remain after they are physically gone.

One thing that I sometimes hear from women when I'm doing seminars is that they are angry at their parents for not providing the kind of nurturing and love that parents are "supposed" to give. There are many advantages to aging. One of the greatest is we have the personal power to give up on what we thought people were supposed to do and the strength to accept what is. You can't change history. What was done is done. If your parents haven't changed by now, chances are they will not. Get over it and move on with your life.

You truly don't need parents anymore, because now you are able to parent yourself, giving yourself the nurturing and love that you need. You now know how to find love in others and are wise enough to understand that genuine love is not bound by blood relationship. You can find deep, life-giving love in many places and from many people. If you have good parents, you get it from them. If not, you can get it elsewhere. In either case, by midlife you have hopefully learned how to find care and support from friends, children, partners, and others. Most of all, you give it to yourself, or can learn to do so.

Friends

One of my dearest friends, Myra, and I were shopping together when I snatched a beautiful, bright plaid blouse off the rack and dashed to the dressing room to try it on. Proud of my find, I came out and modeled it for Myra. Crinkling up her nose, she said, "You look like a picnic table."

That's a true friend, someone who will tell you that you look like lawn furniture when you mistakenly think you look swell. As women age, we tend to develop fewer but deeper friendships than when we were younger. No longer concerned with flitting about in order to be "popular," we spend more time with the women to whom we feel closest and less time with those who are still mired in traditional female competitive games. You know the games I mean, the ones where women try to out-dress, out-man, and outdo one another. Let's face it: One of the things we get tired of in polite society is being polite. With our best friends we are exceedingly kind, extremely supportive, and generously loving, but thank the moon and stars we're not required to be polite. We can gossip outrageously about people we don't like, swear like truckers, and swig down ice cold beer. (Or, as one Southern belle put it, "Swill our iced tea.") Intimate friends are those whom we absolutely trust to never confide our improprieties to another living soul. That's because they are perpetrating the same improprieties.

There's nothing better than having a few intimate friends. If you don't have any, think of how you can start developing genuine camaraderie with others. The best way to begin is by being a true friend.

Communion

Educators Dan P. McAdams and bell hooks [35], (she doesn't use capital letters for her name) talk about "communion." McAdams defines communion as "the overlapping strivings for love, intimacy, interdependence, acceptance, and interpersonal experiences suffused with the emotion of joy" [20]. He distinguishes between love and intimacy, though both are facets of communion.

Love is more complicated because there are so many kinds of love, including erotic love, friendship love, and love of humanity. On the other hand, McAdams says, "To be intimate is to share one's inner self with another. Through sharing, people come to know each other better, and to care for each other" [20]. Intimacy can be a component of and can improve love, but love, especially erotic love (the "hormonal love" discussed earlier) and love of humanity, doesn't always involve intimacy. In one study, McAdams found that there is a strong link between a desire for intimacy at about age thirty and overall happiness seventeen years later in midlife.

In other words, intimacy, even more so than love, leads to contentment in life. Communion, the joining of love and intimacy, entreats us to kneel at the alter of fulfillment as nothing else in life can.

Your Relationships and Your LifeMap

1. Look back at your LifeMap on page 15 and think about the line or absence of a line drawn between your Soul and your Relationships.

2. If there is a connection, are you happy with that connection? _____ If so, what can you do to continue to strengthen the connection? _____

3. If there is a connection but you're not happy with it, what can you do to begin to strengthen that connection?

   _____

4. If there is no connection between your Soul and your Relationships, what can you do *now* to begin to build a connection? (E.g. Get marriage counseling, consider the value of frogs, let go of your grown children, see your parents for who they are, develop intimate friendships, and share communion – love and intimacy – with others and with yourself.)

   _____

   _____

   _____

5. Which one are you going to do *today*?

   _____

6. Visualizing yourself taking care of yourself, especially if you feel like you didn't get the care that a child should get when you were young, can be a meaningful beginning to caring for others. Take some time by yourself, find a spot where you will not be disturbed, sit or lay down so that you are comfortable and do this visualization: *Imagine that you are walking down a nice place, like a favorite street, the beach, or a wooded path. You are alone. As you walk, breathing in the fresh air and enjoying your stride, you see that there is a child coming toward you. As the little one gets closer, you notice that it is a girl. Then you see that it is you when you were a little girl. Observe the look on her face, how she carries her body, and the way that she moves. Is she happy or is she sad? As you come face-to-face you look at her and see all that is there, no longer avoiding the knowledge that lies behind her beautiful eyes. You embrace the girl that is you and make a promise to her that she will never be alone or sad because you, the grown woman, will always be there to take care of her. You will not allow her to be treated poorly and will shelter her from harm. You will love her for the rest of your days. As you hug her, you feel her melt into your body, becoming one with you. Now the promise is one that you have made to yourself. Never forget that the child that is you is within you and that you made a promise to her that you must keep.*

Linda Hughes, Ed.D.

Chapter 7 ~ Your Work

"If you rest, you rust."
Helen Hayes, 1990

My mother, Shirley Hughes Lacey, was an optician for most of her adult life. She loved her work, won a number of professional awards, and was even featured once on television for her skills. She worked in the same office for thirty-five years and had a faithful list of patients who didn't want to deal with anybody but her. But, like most people, she retired when she was 65. There was a big Saturday night retirement party, so my siblings and I traveled from all over the country to join the celebration. There were the traditional toasts, lavish gifts, and lots of food and frivolity. Mom had a great time!

The next Monday morning I called her house to ask how it felt to be free as a bird. There was no answer. On a whim, thinking "surely not," I dialed the office number. She answered the phone.

Using one excuse after another, like somebody was sick or they were especially busy, she worked almost right up until she died nine years later. Retirement just wasn't her style.

The key, I came to realize, to my mom's desire to keep working was that what she did every day was far more than mere work to her. She had deep attachments to her co-workers and patients.

She used her talents and skills to contribute a valuable service to the community. And she loved every minute of it.

Job Satisfaction

Considering that the workplace is where many women spend the majority of their waking hours, a woman's job can't help but play an important role in her life. Studies have shown that work satisfaction correlates with general well-being [36]. In midlife, we tend to shift our focus from being proud of how others perceive our work to being more concerned with how personally meaningful the work is to ourselves. For those who have the option of engaging in meaningful work, that work can contribute to their happiness by providing income, personal satisfaction, social relationships, and a feeling of contribution to others [37]. But, for those who have limited options, real or perceived, work might not contribute to a sense of wellbeing. In fact, the longer a person holds an unsatisfying job, the more likely it will lead to "stagnation" and "refusal to grow" for middle-aged people [27].

Contributing to work dissatisfaction for many midlife women is the reality that, even though they've worked hard for many years, job parity is nowhere in sight. There are societal barriers, like sexism, ageism, and cronyism in our system that prohibit some women from achieving their professional goals [38]. Mix ageism with the wage gap and there's even more disparity for midlife women. "In 1998, women on average earned 76 cents for every dollar a man earned. But women by age 55 earned just 69 cents" [39]. Women are not expected to achieve pay parity until 2050 [39], too late for women who are in midlife at the beginning of the century. Women who are qualified still find it difficult to penetrate that glaring glass ceiling, which former Labor Secretary Alexis Herman referred to as the "cement ceiling" for women of color [39]. Women can become disillusioned, angry, and deflated by such inequities. Laurel Lippert concludes, "Biological, social and psychological factors all affect the quality of the experience a woman has in a particular role" [6]. Thus, a woman's exposure or lack of exposure to unequal treatment can contribute to dissatisfaction or satisfaction with her role as a career woman.

Ask yourself if any of this unequal treatment applies to you. If so, you might not be able to combat all of it, but usually there is something you can do, starting with not selling yourself short. If there's a job you'd like to try for but you're not sure you'll get it, give it a shot. You already don't have that job, so what do you have to lose? Nothing. When it's time for a pay raise, don't be afraid to speak up and ask for what you're worth. You might not get it, but you might get more than you would have otherwise. And when you find people, men and women, who are willing to mentor you and support your professional efforts, accept the offer. Although we're mired in an age-old system that isn't always fair, that doesn't mean there aren't men and women out there who are in positions to help and are willing to do so. Most of them, however, are not psychics – they cannot read your mind. If you want their support, ask for it. If you don't get it, ask someone else. Whatever you do, don't give up.

Selling Yourself

Because there are still prevailing myths about midlife women, like the belief that we're suffering through menopause when in fact most of us are okay, you might have to "sell" yourself for the job that you want. Remember that you've acquired wisdom along the way, wisdom that too many places of employment are missing today. Moreover, midlife women are usually swift learners when it comes to technology, according to LuAnn Cooley, who teaches computer technology. "After all," she says, "we know how to use a keyboard, seeing that we had to take typing in high school in case we were secretaries someday" [40]. Midlife women have good people skills, too. We have to. We've been juggling men, kids, in-laws, neighbors, co-workers, friends, acquaintances and, well, everybody, all of our lives. As a seminar attendee once said, "Anybody who can negotiate who gets the last gummy bear, the 2-year-old or the 9-year-old, can negotiate anything at a business meeting." And, we grew up with values like loyalty and commitment, giving us solid work ethics. The reality is that most midlife women, like you, have valuable skills to offer in the workplace. We're prized employees, so don't let prospective employers get away with thinking you don't have anything to offer.

The Right Career for You

But let's talk about that "workplace" for a moment. If you find that you don't fit into the traditional business setting, maybe it isn't for you. Maybe you're in that line of work because it's what you fell into at some point and maybe there is something else out there that you haven't considered yet. In other words, maybe you are being narrow-minded about the possibilities. That might sound like a switch-back when you read the chapter on money where I suggest that you save for retirement, but if you are unhappy with your career it's possible that you need to consider something else, even if that means making less money. With careful financial planning, you might find that you don't need extras and that you wouldn't mind a different standard of living if it made you more content. People seldom consider planning to make less money, but for some that is what needs to be done. Money doesn't always equal happiness, no matter how many jokes tell us it does.

Your goal is to find and keep a job that makes you happy to go to work, so much so that you might never want to retire. At the same time that you want to aspire to do what is best for you, be realistic. You might never make it to president of the company, but you can find a position that lets you use your best talents and skills. You might not become a billionaire, but you can live comfortably. You might not save the world with your work, but you can contribute to your local community. And then again, you might just do all of those things.

Reinventing Your Career

Interestingly, one study found that the more television a woman watches the more likely she will be dissatisfied with her standard of living, feeling that she doesn't have an exciting enough job and doesn't make enough money to live the lifestyle she deserves [41]. So, the more able you are to do work that is important and meaningful to you, and the less you watch TV, the more likely you'll be satisfied with your work and the more likely that satisfaction will spill over into your sense of wellbeing through midlife and beyond.

One great aspect of midlife is that it is a time of reflection and reinvention, a time when a woman who is not fulfilled in her career is more likely to be motivated to seek another, more satisfying one. If ever you've thought about exploring new occupations, now is the time to do it.

Your Work and Your LifeMap

1. Look back at your LifeMap on page 15 and think about the line or absence of a line drawn between your Soul and your Work.

2. If there is a connection, are you happy with that connection? _____ If so, what can you do to continue to strengthen the connection?

   _____

3. If there is a connection but you're not happy with it, what can you do to begin to strengthen that connection?

   _____

4. If there is no connection between your Soul and your Work, what can you do *now* to begin to build a connection? (E.g. Make a list of what you like about your job, make a list of what you'd like to change about your job, talk to women in other careers that you think you might like, read career planning books, find a career counselor, take a test or survey to see what kind of occupation might fit for you, and try to remember what you always thought you wanted to be when you were a child.)

   _____

   _____

   _____

5. Which one are you going to do *today*?

   _____

6. Visit www.jobhuntersbible.com, the sight of Richard Bolles, who wrote the classic book about careers, *What Color is Your Parachute*, and who is considered to be one of the top career planning experts in the country. On the site you can take surveys to see what occupation best fits you and to connect to job hunting sites.

Chapter 8 ~ Your Money

"We can tell our values by looking at our checkbook stubs."
Gloria Steinem, 1978

What do you spend your money on? That might be any easy question if you don't have much money and do have a lot of children. You know where it goes. You also might know where it goes because you budget and plan the spending of each dime. But for some women money is illusionary, slipping through their fingers and disappearing into the mist. Which type of spender are you?

Taking a long hard look at how you spend your money tells you a lot about yourself. For instance, if you're in debt just buying the basics, you probably need to upgrade your skills and seek better-paying work. If you're in debt because you buy too much junk, ask yourself what "hole" it is inside of you that you're trying to fill with all of that stuff. If you manage money well, give yourself a pat on the back for doing what far too few women do.

Money might seem like an odd topic to talk about in connection with the soul. Yet, if we're not clear about our beliefs and habits regarding money we don't really know ourselves. Understanding this extraordinarily important facet of living in this culture helps us understand our values, beliefs, and habits.

Mucho Mullah

As we age, Baby Boomer women are going to need more money than women in previous generations needed because we'll live longer, with a life expectancy projected to be between 81 to 84 years old. Life expectancy for women today in the U.S. is 79 years; for men it is 74 [42].

In fact, it's estimated that we will need to have $1 million dollars saved in order to live our later years in relative comfort. If you retire at 65 and live for twenty more years, and you're accustomed to $50,000 per year (according to the U.S. Bureau of Labor Statistics the average U.S. household income in 2001 was about $42,000), that's $1 million worth of living. Add to that inflation and increased medical expenses as we age, and a cool mill isn't even enough.

Here's even more depressing news, although I hope that instead of sitting around in a funk you'll get motivated to do something so that you don't become a sad statistic: The average age of widowhood in the U.S. is 56 years old [43]. (The number is so low because young men tend to die in accidents and old men die of age-related causes. So, adding the young to the old produces a younger average than one might expect. I was widowed when I was 28.) Although we wish the statistics were wrong, they aren't and therefore we have to face the reality that the majority of us who are now married will be widowed at some point in our lives. Half of all women over the age of 65 live as widows.

Because of widowhood and divorce, by the year 2020 it is projected that 85 percent of older people living alone will be women. Today 45 percent of women living alone are poor or near-poor, and that number is expected to increase. The reasons are numerous: Women tend to be caregivers to their elder parents, with 75 percent of such care being administered by women. This diminishes their ability to work outside the home and drains their financial resources. Young adult and midlife women are more likely than men to have intermittent careers while they care for their children. Therefore, they are less likely to have their own pension plans. Because they pay less into Social Security, their benefits are less than men's. The average Social Security check for a woman in 2002 was $412 a month. One third of all elder women rely on that check for their sole income [44]. In other words, they live in poverty.

Pish Poor Planning

Do you have a million dollars stowed away? If so, great. But most of us don't. That means we need to start planning now in our middle years so that we won't be living in poverty later on.

There are quick and easy answers about what to do in order to have money in old age:

- ✓ Don't ever retire.
- ✓ Marry well.
- ✓ Make a million with your own business and investing acumen.

✓ Win the lottery.

Those are the answers I hear from some women at seminars. Not very realistic, are they? True, we may not be able or want to retire at 65, but most of us at some point will need to at least slow down. Marrying for money spoils my chapter on relationships, which suggests that you find intimate love. If we all knew how to make our own million, we'd be doing it. And winning the lottery? Forget about it!

Praiseworthy Planning

What is realistic is for each of us women to face the fact that we need to do our own saving for retirement. Don't depend on a husband or someone else to do it for you. If you're single, you already know what I'm talking about because you take care of money for yourself. If you're married and doing this kind of planning with your spouse so that you will both be well cared for, that's good. Make certain, however, that you are actively involved in that planning. You need to know what to do if the time comes that you're taking care of finances by yourself.

I'm often pleasantly surprised by how many women tell me that they do in fact have a good chunk of money set aside for retirement. Many of them are women who work in ordinary jobs every day of their lives, did not inherit money, do not get alimony checks, and have typical family obligations. When I ask them how they managed to save so much, I hear the same answers time and again:

- ✓ Stay on a budget.
- ✓ Don't "shop," only buy what you need.
- ✓ Use discounts and coupons.
- ✓ Set aside a percent of your check every pay period, no matter how difficult.
- ✓ Invest very conservatively.
- ✓ Say "no" to your children when they want everything other children own.
- ✓ Do not fall for "get rich quick" schemes.
- ✓ Drive your car until it drops.

One woman offered this tidbit of advice: If you think you really want to buy something you see in a store, make yourself wait until the next day. Chances are you won't even remember it. Another told of how she could only save $25 a month, but it added up to a nice nest egg. A number of housewives have admitted that they surreptitiously take a percent of the household budget and put it into savings.

Businesswomen Sue Forrest always figures "cost-per-wearing" or "cost-per-use." Let's say you find a $100 scarf that you fall madly in love with and in your delirium you think you can't live without it. How many times are you going to wear that little piece of fabric? Ten times? Well, then Sue says it's too expensive. One hundred divided by ten is ten. That means it costs you ten dollars

84

every time you hang the thing on your neck. She suggests that you *rarely* ever let yourself purchase an item unless you can get it down to $5 per use. Exceptions would be something like the dress you wear as mother of the bride or groom, or your own wedding dress, but not much else.

You'll save yourself a lot of junk in your closet, some heartache, and a chunk of money if you follow simple, practical rules like these. You don't have to be a financial wizard in order to save money. (Have you noticed that some of those bigwig Wall Street guys aren't doing too well, anyway?) Use common sense and do whatever it takes to secure your financial future.

Do It for You

You might fear that it's too late. A little is better than nothing. And you might be surprised if you start now, when you're forty, fifty, or sixty, at how much you can put away in the next ten or twenty years. You probably won't be able to stash a million bucks, but you can make the difference between poverty and moderate comfort in your old age. Best of all, you can keep yourself from having to depend on others, like children or siblings, to take care of you. There's always a chance they won't have the money anyway, so do it for yourself.

Linda Hughes, Ed.D.

Your Money and Your LifeMap

1. Look back at your LifeMap on page 15 and think about the line or absence of a line drawn between your Soul and your Money.

2. If there is a connection, are you happy with that connection? ____ If so, what can you do to continue to strengthen the connection?

   _____

3. If there is a connection but you're not happy with it, what can you do to begin to strengthen that connection?

   _____

4. If there is no connection between your Soul and your Money, what can you do *now* to begin to build a connection? (E.g. Stop shopping, set a budget, save a percent of each paycheck, say "no" to your children's extravagant requests for gifts, figure cost per use, keep your old car, read books and listen to tapes about financial planning, stay away from "get-rich-quick" schemes, and ask advice of people who've proven their ability to handle money well.)

   _____

   _____

   _____

   _____

5. Which one are you going to do *today*?

   _____

6. There are so many books about money that you will have no
trouble finding them in the library or at the bookstore. A few of
my personal favorites are: *The Complete Idiot's Guide to
Investing Like a Pro,* by Edward T. Koch and Debra DeSalvo; *Die
Broke: A Radical Four-Part Financial Plan*, by Stephan Pollan
and Mark Levine; *The Millionaire Next Door: The Surprising
Secrets of America's Wealthy,* by Thomas J. Stanley, Ph.D., and
William D. Danko, Ph.D.; and *The 9 Steps to Financial Freedom:
Practical & Spiritual Steps So You Can Stop Worrying,* by Suze
Orman. If you don't know where to start and if one of these titles
appeals to you, check it out. As you learn more about financial
planning, you'll get better at selecting materials that best fit your
individual financial situation.

Chapter 9 ~ Your Space

"Silence is not a thing we make; it is something into which we enter."
Mother Maribel, 1972

Mother Maribel, who was an accomplished artist and nun, was telling us that silence is always there for us, we simply need to step into it. That's why every woman needs her own space, a place that she can call her own, so that she can enter silence there. It might be a spot in the yard, a corner of a room, a favorite table at a café, a bench in a park, an entire room in your home, or your entire home. It needs to be any place where you can shut out the rest of the world and think your own thoughts. If you're exceptionally good at blocking out external noise, it can even be a public place.

Women have a marvelous way of developing their own rituals in order to find their own space, especially if they are swarmed by other people in their daily lives. I've heard of sitting alone in the junk room at work, pulling off the highway and parking in a pretty spot, meditating while in yoga class, sitting under a tree on top of a hill, praying in church when it's empty, and pretending to nap on the subway train while actually doing a relaxation visualization exercise. The lengths to which women go in order to enter their own worlds of silence, so that they may bring into it only the sounds that they choose, illustrates the need for such silence.

Do you have a space just for you? Mine is the bedroom window that overlooks the backyard. I've set a small wicker table in front of the window, with a tray of candles on top. Each color candle represents something that is sacred to me: blue for peace, red for love, yellow for joy, cream for grace, white for protection, and green for the earth. The candles are surrounded by cherished pebbles that I've brought home from my favorite places all over the world. There's a pillow on the floor for kneeling and a basket on the bottom shelf of the table containing prayer books, matches, and dog treats. Because our dog spends prayer time with me, the treats make sense in my spiritual spot. What makes sense in yours?

You might be thinking that you need direction in deciding what to do with your own space, and there are some good resources, like the chapter about "Women's Alters: Seat of Power" in Mary Faulkner's book, *The Complete Idiot's Guide to Women's Spirituality* [45]. You might find that helpful or you might not want anything like an alter in your space. You might not want anything but space. Only you can decide what's best for you. For example, I decided what I wanted for my space, like my candle colors. They're just made up. I don't know if those colors signify anything to anyone else and it doesn't matter. You, too, can do whatever you choose in your space.

Hearing Your Own Voice in the Silence

The purpose of having your own space and allowing yourself a daily time of silence is so that you will be able to hear your own voice, your own inner thoughts. Not the musings, lessons, complaints, opinions, profundities, snivelings, and dictums that you're bombarded with from others, but your own messages to yourself. In a world swirling with written and verbal information, it's hard to separate ourselves from it all and grasp our own soul's missives. Taking time to be in your own space every day will allow you to do that.

Some people believe that each human soul chooses a life direction before coming to earth. There's the old legend that the dent between your nose and upper lip, the nasal cleft, was put there by God's finger just before you entered this life. He shushed you and reminded you to keep your secret of knowledge of existence beyond earth's domain, until that knowledge could be used in ways that wouldn't frighten others. So, the lore continues, some people forget the purpose they chose for being here and don't become aware of it until later in life. Most of that forgetting is caused by our culture that tells children, when they tell us about their soul's knowledge, that they're imagining things and should stop. Have you ever told a child not to pretend to have an imaginary friend? Have you ever scoffed at a little one's proclamation that she was going to be an astronaut someday? Have you ever stymied a child's creativity so that he would fit into a cultural box in order to make your life more comfortable? Have you ever had that happen to you?

Whether or not you believe that people enter life on earth with a destiny to fulfill, you would probably agree that all of us need to use whatever skills and talents we have in the best ways possible, for our own benefit and for the benefit of others. For instance, if you're a patient, kind, loving person, parenting might be your gift to the world. If you're short-tempered, cranky, and curmudgeonly but can write legal documents like a magician, you need to spare the children and help people stay out of legal trouble instead of parenting.

We all have our own gifts and no one's gift is of more value than another's. All of our skills, talents, and abilities, as long as they are life-giving rather than life-threatening, are of equal value. That means that a young mother who cares for her children is contributing as much as the President of the United States. The difference is that in our culture the mother's daily offerings don't get media attention and the president's do.

How do you find out what are your gifts to give to the world? What if you don't know for sure that you have anything to give? You do, you've just lost touch with it. That's why private time and space are so important, so that you can listen to yourself tell yourself what you need to know. You need to hear your own voice.

Educator Elizabeth Hayes [46] writes that there are three meanings to the word voice: (1) talk, (2) an expression of identity, and (3) a sense of power. Listen to what you say to yourself and consider these meanings. What are the actual words that you talk to yourself with? Are they angry, patient, happy, or sad words? Are they words that will help expand your LifeMap or are they limiting it? What do those words say about how you feel about yourself, about your identity? And does that give you a sense of personal power or does it strip you of power? How does that play into your ability to be effective within your family, workplace, community, country, and world? As women our political power is limited, but no one can take our personal power away from us but us. We must not do so.

Listening to your inner voice will tell you a lot about yourself. If you don't know where to start, consider what you used to say to yourself when you were a child. Think back to that time before cultural constraints bogged you down, that time when you were a wild child, and felt no fear and no limitations. You'd coast down a hill on your bike with wild abandon without ever considering what the wind would do to your hair. You'd climb a tree, scrape your knee, and think that represented a badge of courage instead of fretting that it might get infected. And you'd wear your pink tutu, green swim mask, and red patent leather shoes out in public because those were your favorite things, never worrying about whether or not your appearance was socially acceptable. What did you tell yourself about yourself back then? What were you like? What did you want to be when you grew up?

When I was ten years old I wrote in my diary that I was going to be a "writter" when I grew up. I'm pretty sure I meant writer, but if not there's yet another career out there waiting just for me. What's waiting for you?

If you were an abused child, you might have to think further back than childhood and consider what came before, during that time before God put His finger to your lip. Let your mind stretch into your imagination's outer space and consider possibility. It's possible there was and is a time and place when you could be safe, secure, and happy. It's most likely that time is now.

Throw Out the Space Junk

We all have gifts to give in this life. In order to know what those gifts are, we need to listen to what we say to ourselves. In order to hear ourselves, we each need a place that is our private space. Finding that kind of space might mean you need to throw out some space junk, like physical stuff that clutters your place and mental attitudes that clutter your mind. You need to clear your place and clear your mind so that you can be open to whatever possibilities lie ahead in the vast expanse of your own soul system, the universe of your life.

Your Space and Your LifeMap

1. Look back at your LifeMap on page 15 and think about the line or absence of a line drawn between your Soul and your Space.

2. If there is a connection, are you happy with that connection? ____ If so, what can you do to continue to strengthen the connection? _____ If there is a connection but you're not happy with it, what can you do to begin to strengthen that connection?

   _____

3. If there is no connection between your Soul and your Space, what can you do *now* to begin to build a connection? (E.g. Clear a space at home for sitting in silence, learn to meditate, find a favorite spot out in nature, locate a quiet room at work, go to church during a weekday and pray alone, plan a pretty drive, walk on the beach, and use visualization techniques where you imagine you're someplace else when you're in a crowd.)

   _____

   _____

   _____

4. Which one are you going to do *today*?

   _____

5. Mary Faulkner suggests that if you choose to make a home alter, its purpose is to:

...reflect the things you cherish. An alter works symbolically, giving form to what is sometimes very hard or even impossible to form in words.... Through the process of putting it together, bits of truth and wisdom begin to surface. Later, as you reflect over what you've gathered and placed in your alter, a deeper truth about yourself and the things you hold closest to your heart emerge. [45]

Chapter 10 ~ Your Spirituality

"Spiritual love is a position of standing with one hand extended into the universe and one hand extended into the world, letting ourselves be a conduit for passing energy."
Christina Baldwin, 1990

"Spirituality is not the same as religion," Elizabeth Tisdell, Ph.D., reminds us. "Religion is an organized community of faith that has written codes of regulatory behavior, whereas spirituality is more about one's personal belief and experience of a higher power or higher purpose" [47]. In my study of midlife women, I found that some were able to practice their outside traditional religions while exploring deeper spiritual meaning within themselves. Others were turning their backs on religion while moving toward enhanced spirituality. They found their old churches to be too male-dominated, narrow-minded, and boring. One study participant, Lily, said, "I was in church, the church my husband and I had belonged to for years, and I sat there listening to our same old chauvinistic preacher giving his same old chauvinistic sermon and I just couldn't listen to one more word. I up and quit the church."

In their spiritual quests, women seek more than the same old traditions. In my study, women were looking for and found two primary things when they sought spiritual growth: (1) it helped them make meaning of their lives and of life in general, and (2) spirituality was a springboard for expressing unequivocal hope and happiness. In this chapter I'll review more of what the study participants revealed about their spirituality. Hopefully, their insights will be helpful to you as you explore yours.

Meaning-Making

There's a wonderful theory of adult learning, called transformative learning theory, developed by Dr. Jack Mezirow [48], in which he contends that grown-ups are motivated to learn when they want to make sense of something. Other studies have found that in midlife people don't necessarily want more experiences, they've already had a lot of experiences and now want to make sense of them [27]. In other words, they don't want another cruise, marriage, or career until they make sense of the ones they've had. Put those two concepts together and you have a lot of middle-aged people who are motivated to open their minds and learn so that they can make sense of their lives. Mezirow believes that three conditions allow us to learn in ways that transform our lives: (1) critical reflection about our assumptions, especially those assumptions we've held for years and now suspect could be wrong, (2) rational discourse to examine our beliefs, where we talk over our views with others, and (3) taking action. Mezirow said, "We learn to negotiate and act upon our own purposes, values, feelings, and meanings rather than those we have uncritically assimilated from others – to gain greater control over

ourselves as socially responsible, clear thinking decision makers."
We're ready to give up the meanings that were handed to us when we
were young and ready to make our own.

Making meaning, trying to make sense of life, occurred in two
ways for the women in my study, through the development of new
religious beliefs and by exploring thoughts about death. In some cases
there were epiphanies, unexpected revelatory circumstances that
changed their attitudes overnight, and in other cases, the development
of new beliefs happened quite consciously over long periods of time.

Jonni developed new religious beliefs as she matured and
began reading books about spiritual beliefs that were dramatically
different than those she was raised with. She was raised a Baptist and
then was "forced to join the Church of God" during her first marriage,
of which she said, "Those are good but sad people in my opinion. It
was all fear of Hell and you couldn't do anything that wasn't a sin....
They weren't in touch with reality." By reading Edgar Cayce's books
about reincarnation and by experiencing past-life regressions with a
hypnotherapist, Jonni has come to believe in reincarnation.

Jonni explained:

I believe that everything we do here on earth
influences what we'll need to do in our next lives.
When I started to explore my past lives, they just
seemed to fit so much better than that church stuff... I
know I was a priestess of some sort in an ancient
community. I know I wore a long, white robe and I

was there to help people. And I'm here to help people now.

Jacqueline spoke at length about when she was in her twenties and went to seminary. "It really was a transcendent experience where I was truly living in flow." She continued, "So I learned what a lot of these books [self-help books] talk about…when living what you feel is your call…things literally do cleave to you and from you in ways that you really can't talk about." But she got away from her "flow" and found "the emptiness of that lifestyle," which has motivated her to read and explore in order to rediscover her original calling, redesigning it to fit her life today. Even though she holds a doctorate of divinity degree, she said, "I still have no interest at all in just working with a church or religious group." She says she has "a much more ecumenical approach."

Jacqueline concluded that, "The workplace, maybe the corporate world, may be exactly what I need. Because if anybody needs the message today it's the Worldcoms and Enrons." Her new career as a "life coach" in corporate settings fits her new approach to religion. By using current resources, like popular books on business and spirituality, she is able to teach life skills including "work in ethics, kind of sliding in the spiritual side."

Oceanne has made drastic changes in her religious beliefs. She said that during her midlife changes "my spirit wanted to go higher" and she did a lot of "soul searching." That was easy to do in Atlanta, she said, because "this place is so spiritual." She turned her back on her fundamentalist upbringing and attended a Unity church with "a female that was a minister." Oceanne declared, "I was a different person." She added, "The minister…this was father's day, she went into this meditation of prayer…around being a father-mother God… she was just taking me on a journey about God and who God was and was a more expanded expression of God." Later, Oceanne attended seminars at that church and bought seminar tapes that she would end up playing over-and-over. That's when she had a "fight with God." The result was "I have a much bigger God today than I did at that point…." Her change in beliefs "drew lots of spirituality, lots of people." She's now a member of a women's spiritual group that meets to discuss the spiritual books they have read and other issues; and, she attends a Buddhist community center. She concludes, "I'm fascinated by what I feel now about my spirit."

Rose's grandfather was "a Quaker Preacher…and my grandmother was a healer, a witch." The grandfather was on the paternal side of her family and the grandmother on the maternal side. Rose said, "It was a strange group…I got to watch grandma in the middle of the night. She's the only witch I ever saw that would have a cauldron and a shotgun at the same time." But that grandmother would "go to church. I could not figure out why in the hell she drove me there. And she'd go, 'We have to fit in.' I said, 'I don't.'"

And she hasn't, practicing a variety of religions in her own way. Rose said, "Every religion. I love them all. I think they are all just different belief systems that God has put here on Earth so that man can understand who he is… And so I like the Druids, I like the

Catholics...the Baptists." She continued, "I like all of them, so I use all."

Rose explained, however, that she doesn't need to attend any type of group service. "I've got my own circle in the backyard... I light my candles. I open up the energy. I call in my guardians and have them put in a boundary of protection and I do my work there." She noted, "I don't need to speak to any other person to get my request done. I do a lot of work on different dimensions." Rose continued, "Around thirty-five [years old], something activates and it's like somebody reaches in and flips the switch and says, 'Okay, now you've played around way too long... We are going to start showing you glimpses of a multi-dimensional world." She stated that our "inner knowledge" becomes activated as we age. She noted, "Most of our young adult lifetime, I think, the women in our age, we spend just trying to survive... We have some gifts that we don't even use until we are able."

Lily mentioned "ancient woman-centered religions" that she'd been reading about and said they "open a whole new world." Walker spoke of "the goddess I've become so close to [through reading and meditation], who brings me so much peace." Susan's religious beliefs have expanded to include a bit of humor. She said that God supported her work as a writer some years ago when she tried working as a real estate agent. Smiling, she explained, "God did not want me to be a real estate agent so He gave me psychotic sellers and buyers. They were wonderful material for a book."

Linda Hughes, Ed.D.

The second aspect of meaning-making was exploring thoughts about death. Some women have developed new concepts of death as they have aged. Fiona is "fascinated, for some reason, with TV shows about the pyramids," and with "medical shows about disease." She admits to being drawn to sources with "themes of death." Rose has read books and attended seminars that explain what happens after death. And, Jonni loves her books about reincarnation, like Edgar Cayce's *Story of Karma.*

Fiona said:

But the aging thing and the thing about dying and facing eternity - yes, that has become a predominate thought that I never would have had twenty years ago. Maybe not even ten years ago. But…I'm restructuring my own thoughts about myself and… I begin to think about things like that. What's going to happen? What is death? Is there something after? Is there spiritual? I find myself to be a more, not a spiritual person because I felt I always was in some respect. Not in a traditional sense. But if spiritual can mean more forgiving, kinder, trying to be more thoughtful of others, less interested in myself, then I think I do become that as I get older.

Jonni talked about wanting to get this life right so that when she dies her next life will be "enriched" by this one. "That's a lot better," she said, "then having to learn everything all over again

102

because I didn't pay attention this time. I'm very aware that I only have so much time left to get it right."

Ask yourself if your thoughts about death have increased as you've aged. That doesn't necessarily have to be a morbid thing. It can mean that you, like these women, are thinking more about the meaning of your life and that you want to make the best of it while you're here. In order to accomplish that, you might benefit from exploring new religious practices that will allow your spirituality to open up to possibility.

Hope and Happiness

Meaning-making is the first aspect of spiritual growth, and the second aspect is two-fold: hope and happiness. Psychologist Martin E. P. Seligman, who is a former president of the American Psychological Association, contends that long-term happiness is difficult to recognize, admit, and express in this culture because psychology has for years been drilling into us that we should concentrate on the deficits rather than pluses in our characters. He says that not only do we want positive feelings, we want acknowledgement that we are "entitled to our positive feelings." When we are alienated from positive emotions, he says, it "leads to emptiness, to inauthenticity, to depression, and, as we age, to the gnawing realization that we are fidgeting until we die" [49]. For some women, emptiness, inauthenticity, and depression are trigger events that precipitate their exploration of spirituality.

Supplementing Seligman's theory is educator Carol Gilligan's belief that joy is a difficult emotion for women because, living in a patriarchal society, we have not been taught that it is our right to expect to experience pleasure, happiness, and joy. Gilligan says that women must allow history to fall away and let "life [come] into the room" [50]. Many women have taken the first steps and some have taken leaps (rather joyous ones at that) in freeing themselves from the shackles of the history of societal expectations. Even though they might still be suffering from set-backs and disappointments, they are allowing themselves to be happy on their own terms.

For example, Oceanne said, "I have so many gifts and so many talents now I know that I am truly loved." She learned to feel loved by joining spiritually-based support groups and attending seminars, a far cry from feeling unloved after her divorce years ago.

Fiona professed her happiness, saying, "I have this most wonderful life. A wonderful life. I have people who love me and people I love. ..." Sweetness said, "I am very lucky and I'm very blessed in my life. I have a lovely extended family and friends and my husband is the absolute most wonderful person in the world... I am doing exactly what I want to do." Susan said, "I thank God for everything that I have and... I ask Him to give me opportunities to share His love and I thank Him."

Furthermore, Susan stated:

I just think that we are blessed in this country to have the capacity, the opportunity and the capacity to have seasons in our lives as women where we may be performing one function at one phase in our lives and then we will go into something totally different and what a blessing it is to have the choice to do that.

Eva and Jacqueline expressed hope for the future. Eva explained that her spiritual beliefs support her as she considers changes in her life. She said, "At about [age] fifty-five, I know I'm going to change my life. I don't know what I am going to do yet... But it's going to be good." Jacqueline talked about "redefining her identity." She said, "I feel very hopeful about it. I am working so hard and I'm willing to go into it. I'm real hopeful that I'm going to come out much deeper and richer on the other side of it. But I'm not there yet."

Jacqueline concluded by saying:

I love everything about my life. I am very much in process. I have miles and miles to go. I'm dealing with issues that I have never dealt with before. But, I really do know, I have a peace inside and I really do know I'm on track and moving in the right direction.

So you see that hope and happiness are not always easy to find. But they are there. The trick is to stop sitting around waiting for hope and happiness to find you but for you to go out and find them. Spread your wings and fly until you run smack dab into the middle of them.

"What about Me?"

Right about now you might be wondering what's out there for you in that unexplored space of spiritual growth. You've read these women's stories, heard my rah-rah cheer about hope and happiness, and are saying, "That's great for them, but about me? How does this fit for me?" One thing that we know for sure about spirituality, and there's a lot we don't know, is that it is so intensely personal that no one can answer those questions for you except you. Reflect back on what you just read and ask yourself if your life is enhanced by your present religion, if you practice one, or if you feel stifled by it.

If you're genuinely enriched, that's great. But if, like Lily, you feel disrespected by your church's practices or if, like Oceanne, you feel as if your spirit wants to "go higher," it's time to do some exploring. These women learned about spirituality by reading books, attending spiritually-based support groups, trying out new churches, keeping journals, praying, meditating, watching educational television, talking to others, searching Internet sites, attending seminars, and listening to motivational audiotapes.

Ask yourself if there is a sense of meaning to your life. Do you feel a sense of purpose? If not, it's time again to do some more exploring.

Then ask yourself if you are afraid of or accepting of the reality of eventual death. Do you fear death because you fear that you're wasting your lifetime? Women who feel fulfilled with their lives have accepted death as a reality, even though they don't want to visit it anytime soon. But understanding that our lives here on earth are finite, that life here will indeed have an end, helps us better use the time of life that we have. If you don't even want to hear the word "death," if you're still pretending that it will never happen to you, yes, it's time to do some exploring.

Another question is: Are you happy? Not the yippee-skippy kind of happy that we see in the movies, but deep-down contentment with how you're conducting your life. If not, it's time to do some exploring.

And even if you feel satisfied with your answers to each of these questions, spiritual growth means that you're always moving into new soul territory, always open to what else is out there in the universe that will caress and kiss your soul, and make you feel whole. Tisdell says, "Spirituality...connotes wholeness and what gives meaning and coherence to life" [47].

God or Goddess?

The quest for a sense of spiritual wholeness is common amongst women. In their study of women and religion, Marci McDonald and Sandra Farran describe "the emergence of a new women's spirituality movement that is making itself felt around the world..." [51]. They and others [47, 52-59] are finding that the male-as-God image simply does not resonate for many women today. McDonald and Farran report that "although women's church attendance has more than halved over the past four decades—with only 25 percent now reporting regular attendance at services—60 percent still expressed spiritual needs."

Some believe that when women practice religion they are more interested in the relationships they learn about and build than in learning about or experiencing a process of being more individual, a process which is called individuation. Nicola Slee, Ph.D., reports, "...women's spirituality is essentially relational in character, rooted in a strong sense of connection to others.... This is in contrast to the classic pattern of male development... individuation" [56]. The reason women desire personal power is so that they can use it for the greater good, for connection to others. This calls for the practice of a new kind of religion.

Women are, Tisdell contends, "...moving beyond the religious tradition of their childhood...and reframing the life-enhancing elements...while developing a more meaningful adult spirituality" [47]. The interconnectedness component of spirituality for women concerns connecting with self and others. Daily meditation or prayer are practiced by many women in order to make that spiritual connection. A number of women in seminars have told me about praying to a goddess every day. But they have different concepts of what that goddess is: a dream of what the woman wants to be herself, an image of an ancient goddess, or a real divine entity. In any case, for some the higher power aspect of spirituality has turned away from the image of a male to a more inclusive vision of God as being Goddess, the Mother of all Life.

Poetess Gloria Lawson has an inspiring poem called *I Am Goddess* [60]. It begins:

I am Goddess

A big statement some might say

For me to be Goddess

Is to be a creator of peace in the world

Every moment of every day

Women like the goddess image for the sense of strength it portrays. According to E. Lisbeth Donaldson [54], the new goddess image that women seek entails five interrelated characteristics: (1) a feeling of rebirth, (2) communion with earth and life cycles, (3) a connection to nature, (4) spirituality instead of religion, and (5) personal power.

Tisdell reports that the women in her study connected to the theme of power by disclosing that spirituality is "a way of life that requires attention to the inner world through centering and meditation, but it also requires action in the world" [47]. Spirituality encourages women to take action in their inner and outer worlds. For many, the goddess image best represents those worlds.

The image of a Goddess is fun, timely, and necessary because religious portrayals have been masculine for far too long. It's no wonder that multitudes of women yearn for an opposite ideal. But when the scale is balanced, with the masculine on one side and the

109

feminine on the other, what we have is in the middle, that space where there is no gender. That is the place where we need to be.

Holy Moly

Regardless of what phrase you use, God, Goddess, Lord, Yahweh, Mohammed, Buddha, Confucius, Holy Spirit, Divine One, All Mighty, Collective Consciousness, or something else, it's time to look beyond the confines of simple words. It's time to reach out as far into the universe as you can go to journey beyond the limitations of such narrow concepts. It's time to grasp an understanding of what is holy.

There is no gender in what is holy. Anyone who contends that God is male or female is thinking too small. There is no church or state in what is holy. Anyone who claims that the Holy Spirit is in this church or that one, or in this country or that one, is thinking too small. There is no favoritism in what is holy. Anyone who says that they are the chosen few is thinking way too small. The Divine One is bigger than any of that. It is inside of us and outside of us because it is everywhere. It is everywhere that we can imagine and everywhere that we cannot. It is all things to all people at all times. It is already here. All you need to do is unfurl your soul and it will be there before you.

Glory be to Midlife on the Highest

Clearly, reframing spiritual beliefs, thinking about religion in new ways, is important to a lot of midlife women. I found that even though many of the women in my study began by seeking information in order to work on other issues in their lives, like relationship or aging concerns, they ended up learning about their spirituality. All roads seemed to lead to spiritual growth. Some had not planned on taking that path, nor had they been especially interested in it when they began, but that was where their journey took them. That little jaunt changed their lives.

As Harriet Cohen, Ph.D., says:

As a result of the spiritual transformation process, women's relationship with the Divine deepens, which is expressed internally and externally by…their spiritual beliefs and spiritual practices. Also, their relationship with the larger culture is altered, as are the beliefs they hold about themselves as women in midlife. [61]

Stephanie Marston found that midlife women, regardless of religion, had changed their daily practices as they aged, and "…have one thing in common: Their spirituality is no longer something they devote themselves to only on Sunday….It now encompasses their lives, moment by moment, day by day" [14].

Linda Hughes, Ed.D.

My prayer for you is that your spirituality, like that of so many midlife women, grows as you age. May that growth take you beyond your wildest dreams into a world of meaning, hope, and happiness, a world that is already waiting for you. All you have to do is breeze on into it. As Melody Beattie wrote, "Each moment in time we have it all, even when we think we don't" [33].

Your Spirituality and Your LifeMap

1. Look back at your LifeMap on page 15 and think about the line or absence of a line drawn between your Soul and your Spirituality.

2. If there is a connection, are you happy with that connection? _____ If so, what can you do to continue to strengthen the connection? _____ If there is a connection but you're not happy with it, what can you do to begin to strengthen that connection?

    _____

    _____

3. If there is no connection between your Soul and your Spirituality, what can you do *now* to begin to build a connection? (E.g. Visit a new church, attend a spiritually-based support group, look up related sites on the Internet, read books about spiritual growth, talk to other women who are interested in this topic, listen to motivational tapes, attend seminars, meditate, read magazine articles about spirituality, seek counseling, take a class, and pray.)

    _____

    _____

    _____

    _____

_____

_____

4. Which one are you going to do *today?*

_____

5. Find a small object that you can carry with you every day in your purse, briefcase, or pocket. It can be a relic (something old that you treasure), medallion (like a saint's medal), familiar (replica on an animal), stone, cross, picture, or anything else that has special meaning to you. Keep it near you as a reminder to pray or meditate. Let it give you peace of mind, strength of character, and love in your heart. Every time throughout the day that you lay your eyes or hands on your object, let it awaken in you hope and happiness. Let it help give meaning to your life.

Chapter 11 ~ Your Life List

"Styles, like everything else, change. Style doesn't."
Linda Ellerbee, 1991

Change is the only thing in life that we can depend on. It's the only thing we know for sure will happen sometime in the future. Maybe even within the next moment. Let's face it, without change life would be stagnant, boring, and not worth living. I know, there have been times in your life when boring would have been a relief. But for the most part, change is what keeps us moving on. It keeps us alive!

The following list gives you some things to think about in terms of change in your life. It might be time to change your thinking, change your ways, change your shoes, make change, or just change everything. It might be time to sit down and plan what it is that you need to change, especially after reading the other chapters of this book and plotting out your LifeMap. By now you have a pretty good idea of what needs to be different in order for you to live midlife and beyond to the fullest. This list reviews much of what has been discussed, so it'll seem familiar. First, write your name at the top of the page. On the left-hand side of the list are things that most of us think or do out of habit. We aren't consciously aware of all of these things, although we are alert to others. Compare the left side with the right. Do you see things on the right-hand side of this list that you would like to do instead of its partner on the left? Circle those items on the right. When you do, you have goals for beginning to make changes. Changes that only you can make.

There's room to add your own comparisons to the list. You might not want to do this all at once, instead mulling it over for awhile. Take as long as you need to do the whole thing, but start with at least one change now. Chawing on it forever belongs on the left side of the page; taking action is on the right.

_____'s Life List

1. Fantasy vs. Reality
2. Blind faith vs. Enlightened faith
3. Wishful thinking vs. Actionable planning
4. Barbie image vs. Health
5. Rumination vs. Reflection
6. Ideals vs. Ideas
7. Self-destruction vs. Self-determination
8. Narrow-mindedness vs. Open-mindedness
9. Hormonal passion vs. Intentional passion
10. Secular vs. Sacred
11. Rules vs. Relationships
12. Logic vs. Intuition
13. Religion vs. Spirituality
14. Spendthrift vs. Thrifty
15. Self-loathing vs. Self-accepting
16. Non-commitment vs. Communion
17. Individuation vs. Connection
18. _____ vs. _____
19. _____ vs. _____
20. _____ vs. _____
21. _____ vs. _____

Did this list make you uncomfortable or comfortable? Would you have to admit that most of what you're doing is on the left-hand side of the list? Or do you feel good that most of what you do is on the right?

If you feel that you'd like to do more of what's on the right but don't know how, read the previous chapters again, find references from the list in the back of the book, or talk to someone. Notice #17 on the list, individuation, thinking you need to be autonomous, versus connection to others. There are qualified people out there who are willing to help you, like a spiritual advisor, friend, support group member, or counselor. They can help you figure out where to begin making positive changes in your life. Wherever it is, begin now. It isn't too late. You're in midlife, which means that you have half of your life left to live.

Chapter 12 ~ Your LifeMap is Your Life

"The real trick is to stay alive as long as you live."
Ann Landers, 1961

As you've read this book, you haven't just been considering how to make a LifeMap. You've been considering how to make a life. The life that you want. The one that you suspected when you were a child; the one that you are meant to live.

You've been thinking about how your body, mind, relationships, work, money, space, and spirituality relate to your soul. You've been thinking about the direction in which you want your life to go. Given that each of us is meant to give our best to this life, hopefully your LifeMap gives you direction so that you know more about what it is that you're meant to give and how you want to give it for the benefit of yourself and others.

Although this book concentrates on what you can do for yourself, other people end up profiting in countless ways. When you're healthier, more mindful, working on good relationships, enjoying your career, secure about money, calm in your own space, and spiritually sound, you can't help but influence others in good ways. If nothing else, you set a good example.

Changes

No one was brought to this earth to be unloved or sorrowful. We pray for those who are and thank the Holy Spirit that we're in a place where we can change that for ourselves should it happen to us.

And we can make those changes. You've always heard that you can do anything you set out to do. You've always heard that because it's true.

When you set out to do something new the end result isn't always what you expected. It can be disappointing or it can be a trillion times better than you ever imagined. Either way, it motivates you to go on exploring your universe until the day you die. And probably after that.

Sometimes when you set out to do something new and you're all excited about it, other people in your life aren't happy about it at all. They don't want you to change. They know you the way that you are. If you change, they'll have to pay attention and get to know you again. That means they'll have to change, too.

It can be so annoying when this happens, but think about it. They aren't in the exact same spot in the universe as you are because no one can be. That means they can't possibly see things from your precise point of view. They haven't had the same experiences and feelings. They're not you. So, be patient. Give them time to make their own changes in their own ways. They might choose never to do that and you might want to make some important decisions regarding that at a later time. But it isn't fair to insist that others think and feel exactly what you are at the moment that you are. They have a right to their own thoughts and feelings, just like you do.

Let me give you a good example. When Lily left her church, her husband didn't understand at first. He was comfortable in that church. As a man, the pastor had never offended him. So Lily didn't insist that he quit, too. She simply went on her own way. Eventually he started asking questions about her new goddess beliefs, which he found bizarre. They went through a period of time when they didn't discuss it. Then he asked more questions and became more comfortable with the change within her. After long consideration, he could understand why she feels the way that she does. He still belongs to the old church, but respects her new practices.

Be patient. Give others time to adjust to changes, especially drastic ones. Other people might never completely understand your decisions, but they can learn to respect your right to make those decisions.

Review Your LifeMap

Look back at your LifeMap on page 15. Read again about the myths that you want to write for yourself in your life. You want to dispel popular myths and be able to say no to depression, no to ailments, and yes to sex. What notes do you need to make or pictures do you need to draw to make sure that your myths, your new personal stories, are on your LifeMap?

Now review the end of each chapter. What are the changes you promised yourself that you'd do *today*? Draw those things on your LifeMap. Extend lines out from each area and write in the good things that you're doing and those that you intend to do. In my seminars, women write those two things in different colors so that they can see the difference between what they're doing and what they need to do.

For example, you might draw two lines out from the "Relationship" circle, one black and one red. At the end of the black line you write "Intimacy," signifying your unconditional love for your child. In red you write "Communion," reminding yourself that you'd like more of an overlap in your life of love, intimacy, interdependence, and acceptance from yourself and others. This is the one you want to work on in order to live your life to the fullest.

In the seminars, each woman gets a large sheet of colored construction paper to draw her LifeMap, so making extensions is easier. You might want to do that, too. A graphic artist once drew an awesome illustration for hers and an artist once went home and painted hers on canvas. If you have that kind of talent, it might be really fun to use it on your LifeMap.

But for most of us our LifeMaps are quite rudimentary. That's okay. As long as they give us a visual reference point, we can take action to do the rest.

No Turning Back

In the oft quoted article titled *Seize the Day, Hour, Minute* from Erma Bombeck's syndicated column, Erma wrote, "If I had my life to live over again I would have waxed less and listened more...I would have eaten popcorn in the 'good' living room...I would have taken the time to listen to my grandfather ramble about his youth...There would have been more I love yous" [62].

Do you ever think about if you had your life to live over? At the end of your life you want no regrets. Use your LifeMap to seize your days, hours, and minutes.

Your goal is to have a Soul System that is in as much balance as possible so that you can appreciate and fully live each moment of every day. Oh yes, like a meteorite hitting your home, there will always be unexpected mishaps. Some will only sting a little and some will temporarily demolish your life, until you rebuild from the strength you have garnered through thoughtful living. And, of course, there will still be some weird aliens roaming in and out of your space, keeping things interesting. But for the most part, your Soul System can bring you extraordinary joy if you let it. That's why taking care of your Soul, taking care of yourself, is so important.

If you're still not certain about how to use your LifeMap to take care of your soul, or just don't know what to do next, start at page 1 and read this book again. It might take a few sittings to get a good grasp on what you want to do. It might even take a few sittings to decide that you're already going in the right direction and want to continue your course.

Midlife Madness

Midlife is often feared when one is younger. It's seen as the beginning of the end. But when we get to midlife we discover that it is the end of nothing and the beginning of a new phase of life that brings with it the possibility for inestimable happiness. We don't lose who we are or what we've been, we simply expand our worlds so that we become more. We become better. That's why so many women claim that this is the best time of life!

This is an exciting time to be at this age. Old midlife myths are falling away to fact; old constraints about aging are crumbling; and, most of us are learning better than to believe that we have to follow someone else's map for our future. We now know that we can chart our own.

As Stephanie Marston wrote:

This is a revolutionary idea, one that goes against the dominant culture. We...no longer have to go along with the game. We're grown women. And by the sheer magnitude of our numbers, we can invent a New Middle Age. Consequently, we can redefine the rules for aging. [14]

Part of what's so exciting about being a Baby Boomer midlife woman is that there are so many of us. As Marston suggested, just by sheer numbers we can change the game. We can chart our own courses. We can let our LifeMaps take us anywhere we want to go.

Life as a Dance

Whew! All of this LifeMapping is pretty serious stuff. Lest you become overwhelmed with the profundity of it all, now that you've done the initial work you deserve a break from your efforts. Take a few moments to imagine yourself journeying through your universe. But how are you traveling through it? Floating is nice sometimes, but that's rather non-action oriented. Flying is good, implying more activity, but it's not quite there yet. How about dancing? One thing that most of us Baby Boomers know how to do is dance. Seeing that we're making up the rules, anyway, why not dance through space? Picture yourself letting go and boogying around your soul system. There's an ancient saying that life is a dance. Dancer Martha Graham said, "Dance is the hidden language of the soul," and choreographer Agnes de Mille said, "The truest expression of a people is in its dances and its music." Think back on the visual image of your life as a universe. Imagine yourself dancing through space, not tethered to earth, not bound by gravity, and not tied to old constraints. Light and free and full of glee. You're not just moving through space, you're dancing through space!

I love the imagery of jiving through our universe, sharing our joy with loved ones, friends, acquaintances, and strangers. It can be any kind of dance. Slow sometimes, rollicking sometimes, but always full of life, showing others that life need not be restrained or dull. It can be this most simple yet most profound thing, this dance of the universe.

I Hope You Dance, the beautiful song recorded by Lee Ann Womack, reminds us, "Never lose your sense of wonder" and "get your fill to eat but never lose that hunger." It asks that we give faith a "fighting chance" and "when you get the choice to sit it out or dance – I hope you dance. I hope you dance" [63].

I hope you do.

References

1. *Webmaster, What is a mandala? 2002, Mandala Project.*
2. *Duerk, J., Circle of stones: Woman's journey to herself. 1999, Philadelphia: Innisfree Press.*
3. *Wall, S. and H. Arden, Wisdomkeepers: Meeting with Native American spiritual elders. 1990, Hillsboro, OR: Beyond Words Publishing.*
4. *Corey, M. and G. Ochoa, Dictionary of film quotations. 1995, New York: Three Rivers Press.*
5. *Hesselbein, F. and J. Collins, Hesselbein on leadership. 2002, San Francisco: Jossey-Bass.*
6. *Lippert, L., Women at midlife: Implications for theories of women's adult development. Journal of Counseling and Development, 1997. 78: p. 16-22.*
7. *Sargent, A.G. and N.K. Schlossberg, Managing adult transitions. Training and Development Journal, 1988. 42(12): p. 58-60.*
8. *McQuaide, S., Women at midlife. Social Work, 1998. 43(1): p. 21-31.*
9. *Gilligan, C., In a different voice: Psychological theory and women's development. 1993, Cambridge, MA: Harvard University Press.*
10. *Hayes, E. and D.D. Flannery, eds. Women as learners: The significance of gender in adult learning. 2000, Jossey-Bass: San Francisco.*
11. *Tisdell, E.J., Feminist pedagogies, in Women as learners: The significance of gender in adult learning, E. Hayes and D.D. Flannery, Editors. 2000, Jossey-Bass: San Francisco.*
12. *Northrup, C., M.D., The wisdom of menopause: Creating physical and emotional health and healing during the change. 2001, New York: Bantam Books.*
13. *Bloch, A., Self-awareness during the menopause. Maturitas, 2002. 41(1): p. 61-68.*
14. *Marston, S., If not now, when? Reclaiming ourselves at midlife. 2001, New York: Warner Books.*

Linda Hughes, Ed.D.

15. Hughes, L., *The role of pop culture in the self-development of midlife women, in Adult Education. 2003, University of Georgia: Athens, GA.*

16. Goode, E., *Antidepressants lift clouds, but lose 'miracle drug" label, in The New York Times. June 30, 2002: New York.*

17. Genazzani, A.R., et al., *Menopause, depression, and plasma opioids. Advanced Biochem Psychopharmacol, 1982. 32: p. 341-346.*

18. Martin, R., M.D., *in Atlanta ABC News. June 28, 2002: Atlanta.*

19. Dowd, M., *Aloft on bozoloft, in The New York Times. July 3, 2002: New York.*

20. McAdams, D.P., *The stories we live by: Personal myths and the making of the self. 1993, New York: The Guilford Press.*

21. Moore, T., *Care of the soul: A guide for cultivating depth and sacredness in everyday life. 1992, New York: HarperCollins.*

22. Hillman, J., *The soul's code: In search of character and calling. 1997, New York, NY: Warner Books.*

23. McCrum, R., W. Cran, and R. MacNeil, *The story of English. 1986, New York: Penguin Books.*

24. Turner, S.L. and H. Hamilton, *The influence of fashion magazines on the body image satisfaction. Adolescence, 1997. 32(127): p. 603-615.*

25. Wolszon, L.R., *Women's body image theory and research. American Behavioral Scientist, 1998. 41(4): p. 542-558.*

26. Hurd, L.C., *Older women's body image and embodied experience: An exploration. Journal of Women and Aging, 2000. 12(3/4): p. 77-91.*

27. Bergquist, W.H., E.M. Greenberg, and G.A. Klaum, *In our fifties: Voices of men and women reinventing their lives. 1993, San Francisco: Jossey-Bass.*

28. Walsh, J., *Study bids good riddance to high heels, in New York Times. 1999: New York. p. 6.*

29. Williams, S., *Heels sock knees, in Newsweek. 1998. p. 72.*

30. Merriam, S.B. and R.S. Caffarella, *Learning in adulthood. 1999, San Francisco, CA: Jossey-Bass.*

31. Gardner, H., *Multiple intelligences: The theory in practice. 1993, New York: Basic Books.*

32. Bateson, M.C., *Composing a life. 1989, New York: Plume.*

33. West, J., in *New Beacon Book of Quotations by Women*, R. Maggio, Editor. 1969, Beacon Press: Boston.

34. Fulghum, R., *It was on fire when I lay down on it*. 1993, New York: Ivy Books.

35. hooks, b., *Communion: The female search for love*. 2002, New York: William Morrow and Co.

36. Merriam, S.B. and M.C. Clark, *Lifelines: Patterns of work and love*. 1991, San Francisco: Jossey-Bass.

37. Mor-Barak, M.E., *The meaning of work for older adults seeking employment: The generativity factor. International Journal of Aging and Human Development*, 1995. *41(4): p. 325-344.*

38. Cunningham, P., *Race, gender, class, and the practice of adult education in the U.S.*, in *Towards a transformative political economy of adult education: Theoretical and practical challenges*, P. Wangoola and F. Youngman, Editors. 1996, LEPS Press, Northern Illinois University: DeKalb, IL. p. 139-160.

39. Glasheen, L.K. and S.L. Crowley, *More women in the driver's seat: But barriers hinder many in midcareer*. 1999, American Association of Retired People.

40. Cooley, L., L. Hughes, Editor. 2001: Buford, GA.

41. Sirgy, M.J., et al., *Does television viewership play a role in the perception of quality of life? Journal of Advertising*, 1998. *27(1).*

42. Census Bureau, U.S., *Population estimates*. 2001.

43. University, T.W.s., *Aging*. 2003.

44. Site, S., *The seniors' site*. 2002.

45. Faulkner, M., *The complete idiot's guide to women's spirituality*. 2002, Indianapolis: Alpha.

46. Hayes, E., *Voice*, in *Women as learners: The significance of gender in adult learning*, E. Hayes and D.D. Flannery, Editors. 2000, Jossey-Bass: San Francisco.

47. Tisdell, E.J., *Spirituality and emancipatory adult education in women adult educators for social change. Adult Education Quarterly*, 2000. *50(4): p. 308-336.*

48. Mezirow, J., *Contemporary paradigms in learning. Adult Education Quarterly*, 1996. *46(3): p. 158-173.*

Linda Hughes, Ed.D.

49. Seligman, M.E.P., *Authentic happiness; Using the new positive psychology to realize your potential for lasting fulfillment.* 2002, New York: Free Press.
50. Gilligan, C., *The birth of pleasure.* 2002, New York: Alfred A. Knopf.
51. McDonald, M. and S. Farran, *Is God a woman? Maclean's,* 1996. **109**(15): p. 46-52.
52. Williamson, M., *A woman's worth.* 1993, New York: Random House.
53. Spellmeyer, K., *Specialists with spirit: new age religion, English studies, and the 'somatic turn'. Religion and the Arts,* 1999. **3**(2): p. 195-214.
54. Donaldson, E.L., *Imaging women's spirituality. Comparative Education Review,* 1996. **40**(2): p. 194-205.
55. Keshgegian, F.A. and N. Baer, *The practice of women's spirituality in 'web' with respect to ritual space. Journal of Feminist Studies in Religion,* 2000. **16**(2): p. 133-148.
56. Slee, N., *Apophatic faithing in women's spirituality. British Journal of Theological Education,* 2001. **11**(2): p. 23-38.
57. Powers, R., *A class that changes lives. Women & Therapy,* 1995. **16**(2/3): p. 175-184.
58. Lauver, D.R., *Commonalities in women's spirituality and women's health. Advances in Nursing Science,* 2000. **22**(3): p. 76-89.
59. Lesher, R., *Litany for soul 2 soul II worship. Journal of Women and Relition,* 2000. **18**: p. 15-17.
60. Lawson, G.J., *I am goddess, in Prelude: A demonstration of life.* 2000, Four Rooms Publishing Company: Fayetteville, GA.
61. Cohen, H.L., *The nature of spiritual transformation for women in midlife, in Department of Education.* 2001, University of Georgia: Athens, GA. p. 266.
62. Bombeck, E., *Seize the day, hour, minute, in Syndicated Column.*
63. Sanders, M.D. and T. Sillers, *I hope you dance.* 2000, Nashville: Rutledge Hill Press.

About the Author

Linda Hughes, Ed.D., is a top-rated motivational speaker and award-winning author who researched midlife women for her Doctorate Degree in Adult Education at the University of Georgia. She is a member of the International Honor Society.

For twenty years Dr. Hughes has worked with tens of thousands of women in this country and abroad presenting seminars and speeches on topics ranging from leadership to life balance. Her *LifeMaps for Women* seminar has long been a favorite and the new version, *LifeMaps for Midlife Women,* has quickly become a hit. Her experiences with over 2000 audiences, as well as her research, afford her a unique and informed perspective on midlife women.

Printed in the United States
18267LVS00003B/316

9 781410 796035